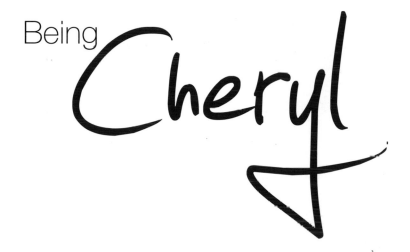

Being Cheryl

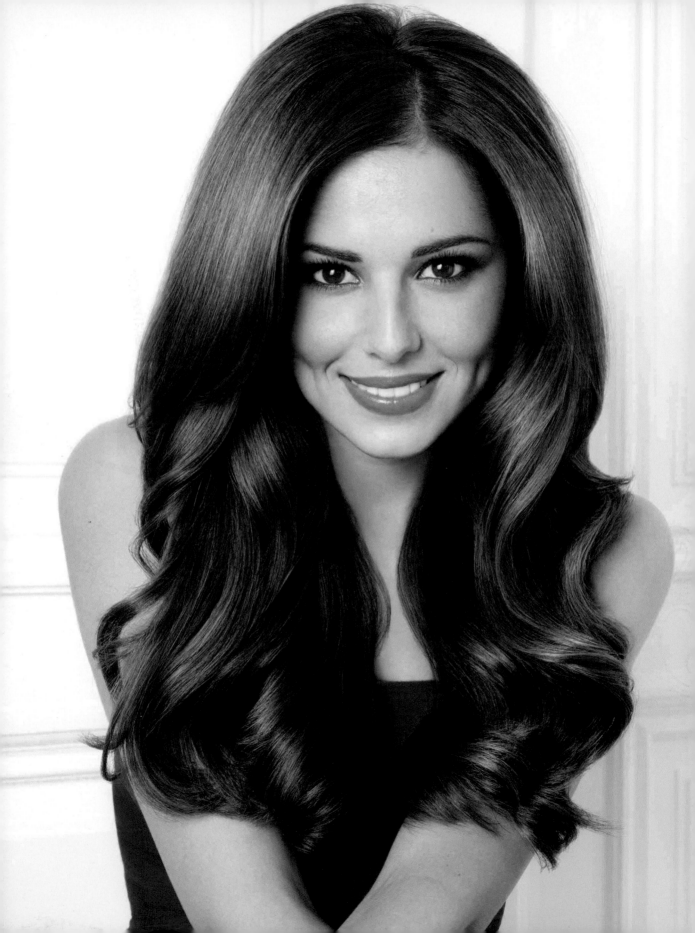

Being Cheryl

Jo Edwards

Illustrated by Nellie Ryan

Michael O'Mara Books Limited

First published in Great Britain in 2010 by

Michael O'Mara Books Limited

9 Lion Yard

Tremadoc Road

London SW4 7NQ

A CIP catalogue record for this book is available from the British Library.

This book has not been approved, licensed or endorsed by Cheryl or her management.

Papers used by Michael O'Mara Books Limited are natural, recyclable products made from wood grown in sustainable forests. The manufacturing processes conform to the environmental regulations of the country of origin.

ISBN: 978-1-84317-501-8

1 3 5 7 9 10 8 6 4 2

Designed and typeset by Ana Bjezancevic

Cover design by Joanna Wood

Printed and bound in Italy by L.E.G.O.

www.mombooks.com

Contents

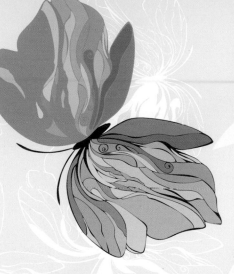

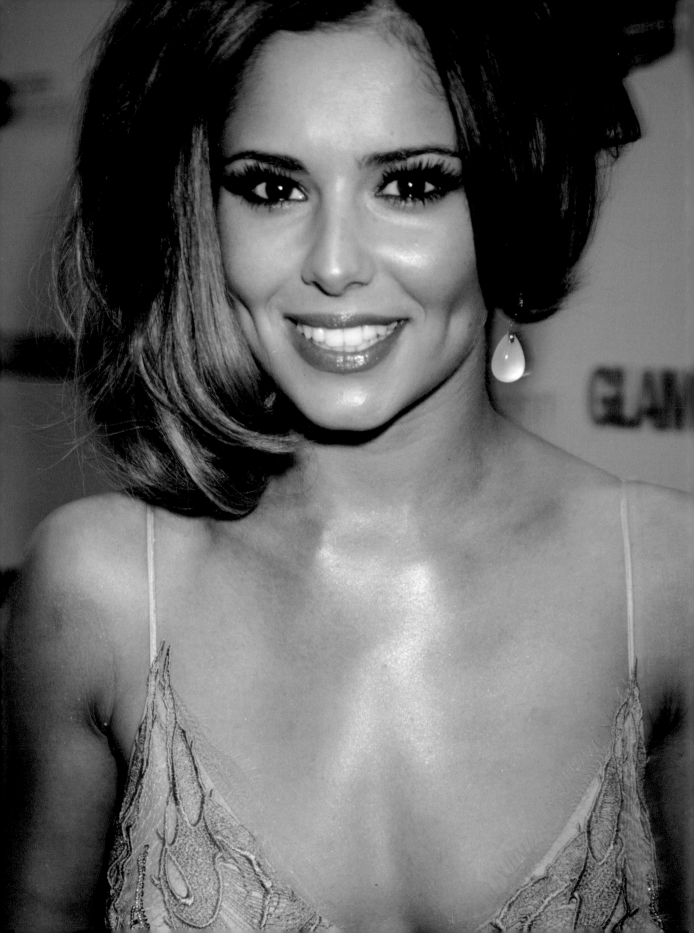

Introduction

Ever since she first stepped into the limelight on *Popstars: The Rivals* – looking unpolished but beautiful, and singing in a voice that quivered with nerves – Cheryl has grabbed our attention.

At first, no one was sure what to make of her; they just knew they were interested in the doe-eyed girl with attitude, who was portrayed as a tough cookie, but who always seemed a more sensitive soul.

But then, as the slashed BacoFoil outfits and clumsy blonde highlights of Girls Aloud: the early years made way for couture and grade-A grooming, and Cheryl emerged from pop-group anonymity to solo stardom, she found her voice – and the nation found a new sweetheart.

'People see me as a role model, but I want them to see I'm human.' *Mirror*

AN ORIGINAL HEROINE

For those of us who are sick of brash and trashy stars – but also tired of media-trained bores, who mouth safe and pre-polished statements – Cheryl has become the new poster girl for glamour, sass, talent and hard work.

The anxious little girl from Newcastle has grown into a polished and poised woman, and now everyone wants a slice of her.

CHERYL'S SECRETS

Cheryl has been immortalized in a pop-art version of the Angel of the North, and her face has become so iconic that it's now printed on cans of hairspray across the country ... but what about the girl behind the big hair, lashes and smile? When she has wiped away the *X Factor* tears and studio gloss, what happens when the cameras stop rolling and she goes home? What does she get up to behind closed doors? Who does she trust?

All the secrets are right here. Discover her beauty routine, her make-up tips, and the style savviness that epitomizes Cheryl. Take a walk in her shoes – along the beach in the Seychelles, into the recording studio, through the backstage corridor of *The X Factor*. Join her for a girlie night out.

This is life, but not as you may know it. This is life with a distinctly Cheryl flavour.

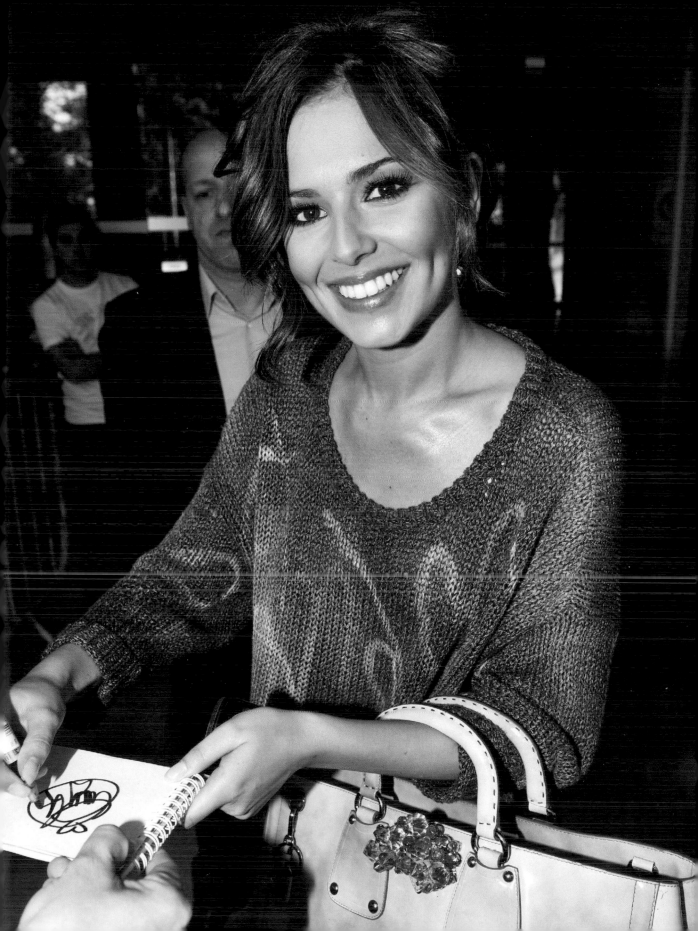

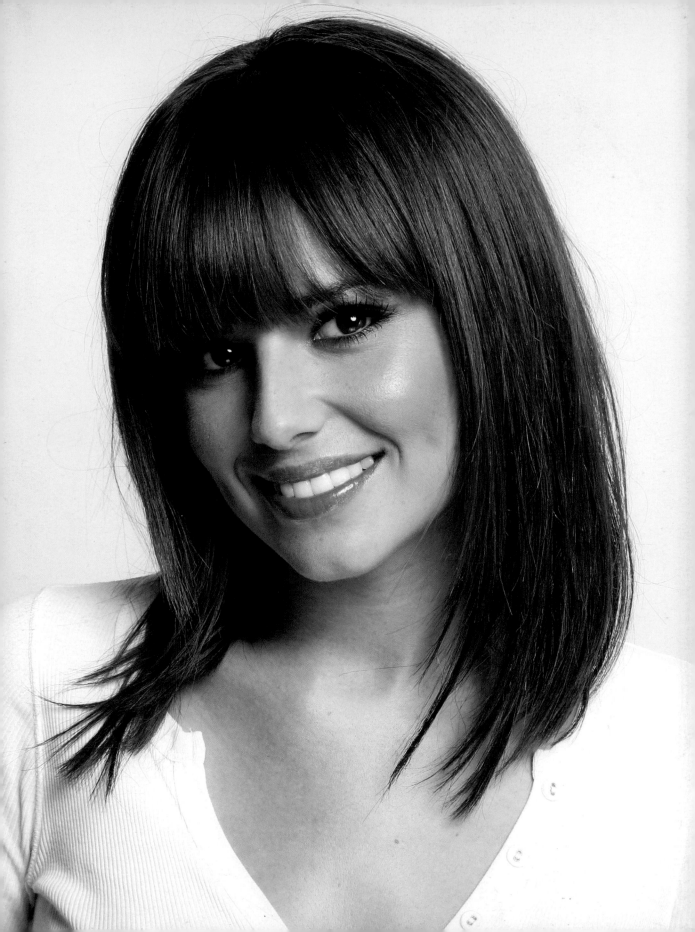

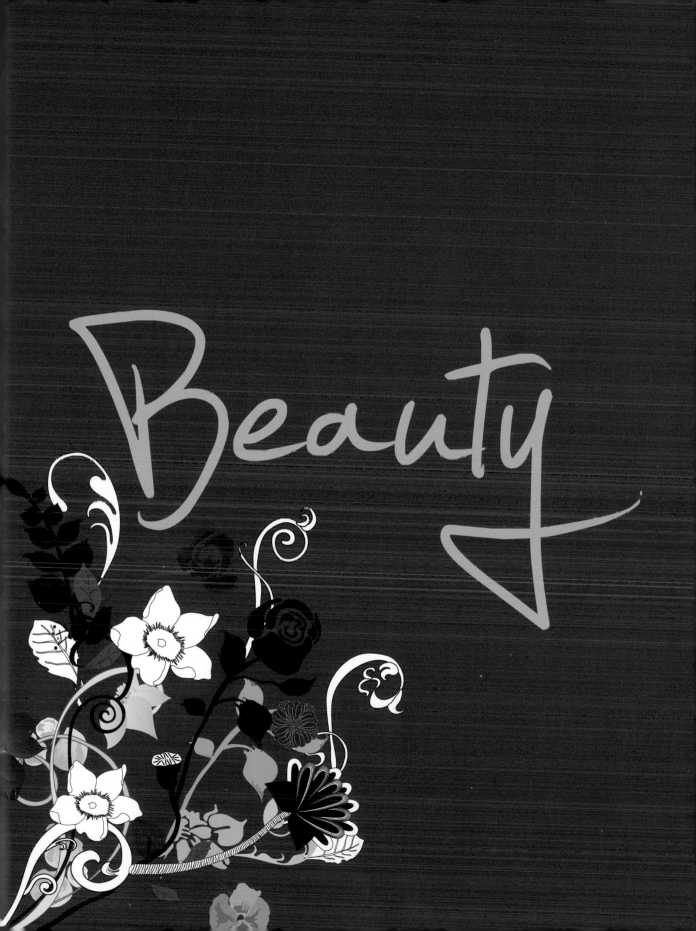

If the outpourings of newspapers and magazines were contemporary poetry, then Cheryl has had countless tabloid sonnets breathlessly bashed out daily on every aspect of her physical beauty.

From her hair ('sparkling chestnut' – *Marie Claire*) to her eyes ('pools of molten brown' – *Harper's Bazaar*) to her smile ('medical balm' – *Vogue*), no feature has escaped fulsome praise from the press. Of course, it helps if you have been smiled upon by Mother Nature, but as all women know, Mother isn't always right and best features can be accentuated, and imperfections played down.

Even though Cheryl is now a hugely successful pop star and Saturday night prime-time princess – who could afford the best of everything in a quest for physical perfection – she hasn't changed much from when she first came into the public eye and remains down to earth ... and that goes for her beauty routines too.

When she closes the doors of her home, washes off the greasepaint and ties her hair off her face, she is still simply Cheryl from Newcastle, using products that can be bought from Boots – she's just got her face on the packaging now.

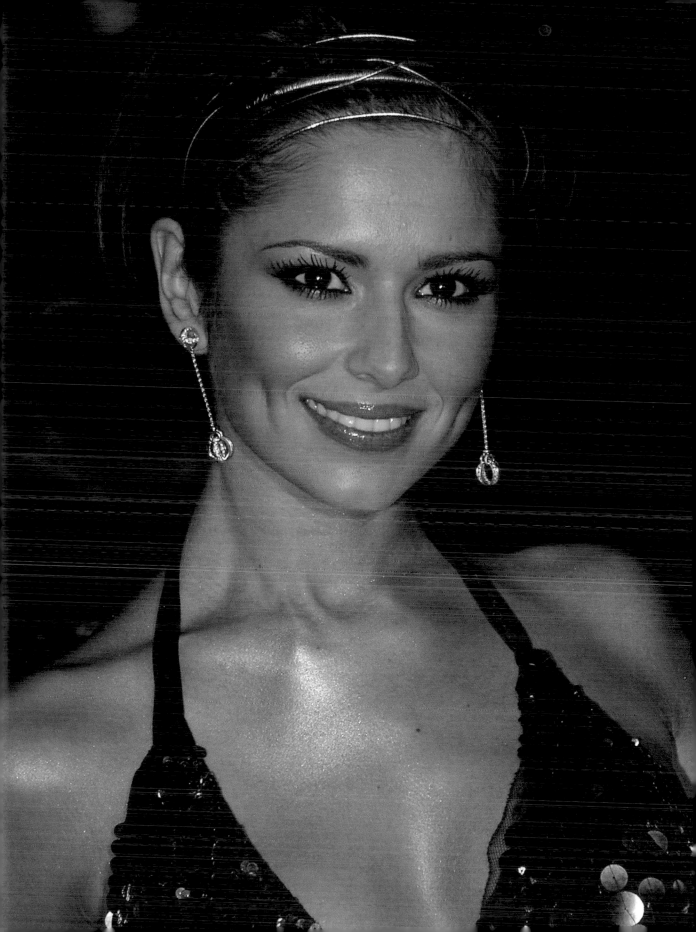

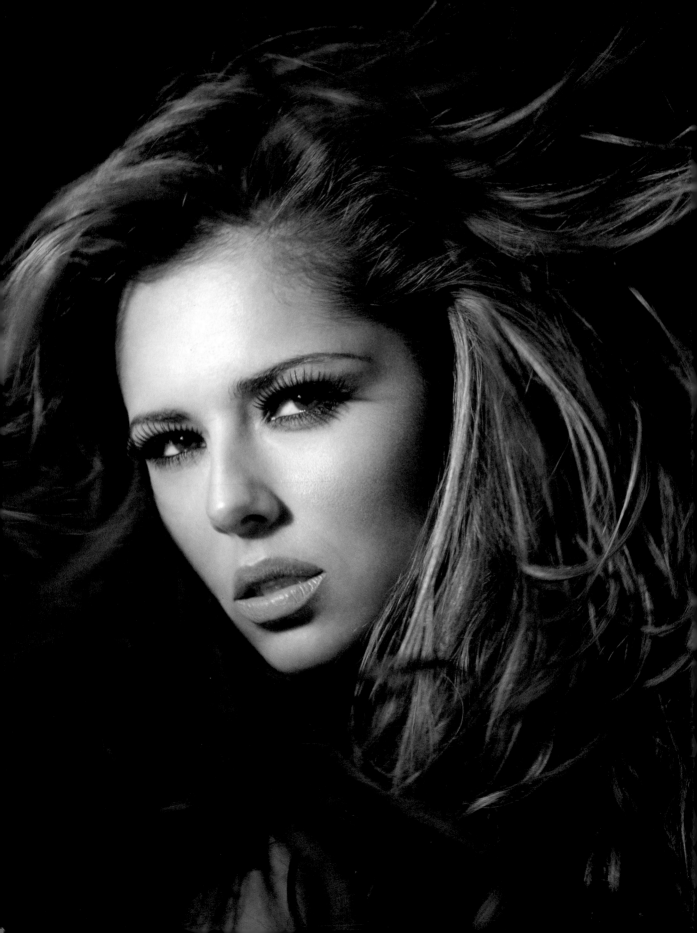

THE HAIR

Many famous beauties have a trademark that is so representative of them, it becomes iconic – Marilyn Monroe had her beauty spot, Elizabeth Taylor has her violet eyes, and so it has become that Cheryl has her glossy mane of hair.

Not since Jennifer Aniston's 'Rachel' cut in the 1990s has someone's hair been so scrutinized, rhapsodized about and mimicked, and yet as Cheryl's fame has grown, so too has the fascination with her tumbling chestnut locks – whether she wears them longer or shorter.

Hair stylist Andrew Barton told the *Mirror*, 'Cheryl's hair is fantastic and fully deserving of style-icon status. The volume she achieves is amazing and makes her hair look glamorous and sexy. Girls love Cheryl's hair so much because it always looks shiny, healthy, luscious and thick. Above all, it is always perfectly groomed.'

Meanwhile, Cheryl told the *Mirror,* 'When my hair looks good, I feel good too. It's my safety blanket and I feel glam when it's long and full of volume. When I'm being styled, I always say, "Make it bigger! Bigger!"'

'My long hair is a blanket for security … If I cut it off, I'd feel like I'd assaulted myself.'

The Times

THE X-TENSION FACTOR

Whether Cheryl opts for the mermaid-length tresses she is most often associated with, or the shoulder-length style she is also fond of, she makes the most of hair extensions – using them not only to add length, but also volume.

The man behind the mane is Julien Guyonnet, who boosts her lustrous locks with monofibre acrylic hair extensions. Julien told the *Daily Mail* online, 'Cheryl has wavy extensions to give her volume. She comes in once every three months for the extensions, and every six weeks for a tidy-up.'

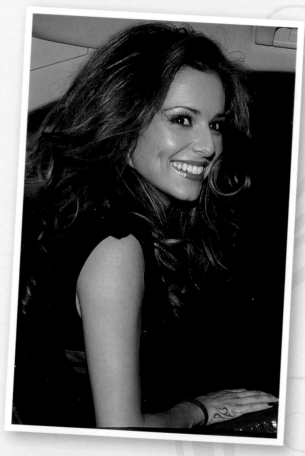

'The higher the hair, the closer to heaven.' *Stylist*

Monofibre has taken over as the preferred choice to human hair extensions as it's lighter and shinier, and is non-porous so it doesn't absorb products, but will hold a particular style.

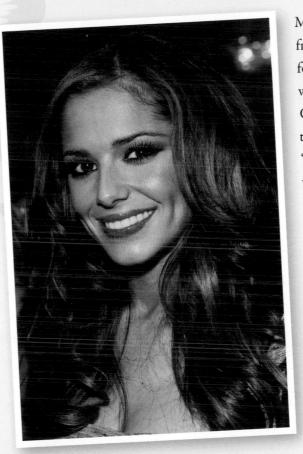

Monofibre extensions cost from £375 and take around four hours to attach. For those who can't afford the price tag, Cheryl has an effective tip, telling fans in a live web chat, 'Tip your hair upside down when you're drying it for volume.' She also recommends using hairspray to boost volume, telling *Stylist*, 'If you want big hair, spray on Elnett then brush it out.' Cheryl advises conditioning treatments to keep locks in tip-top condition, revealing to *Stylist*: 'I always put a hair mask on every couple of weeks.'

'If you're having a bad hair day, forget everything. Stay at home.' *Celebs on Sunday*

TO DYE FOR

Like most girls, Cheryl has not always been kind to her tresses and is the first to admit some style-choice faux pas when she was growing up. She's come a long way from the cornrows, red chunks and peroxide streaks she favoured during her early days in Girls Aloud, but even before that she suffered the odd hair howler.

She told *Hello!* magazine, 'When I was fifteen, I wanted to go peroxide blonde and I spent eight hours in the hairdresser's chair having really strong peroxide used on my hair. I ended up looking like something out of *The Wizard of Oz*, it was awful.'

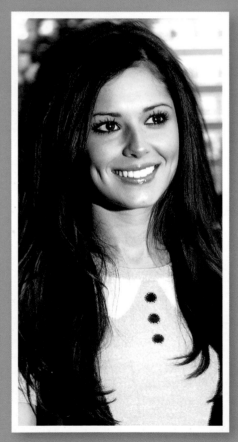

Later, she successfully embraced the use of colour to enhance her locks, dabbling with honey blonde and flirting with a burgundy tint. In autumn 2009, *The Guardian*'s fashion critic Simon Chilvers praised her shade savvy, saying, 'Cheryl has updated her hair shade with a sparky russet. It's a little dangerous, and a trifle high-school gothic, in a sort of *Twilight* way.'

No matter if she experiments with tints, highlights or fringes, she is a true girlie girl and one thing she assures us that she will never go for is a short crop, telling *The Times*, 'I'm not brave enough. It got cut short by accident when I was a kid and I felt violated!'

PROMO PRINCESS

Cheryl found her hairstyle stride in her mid-twenties when, along with her Girls Aloud bandmates, she was signed to promote first nu:u products and then a Sunsilk hair-care range.

All of it was good training for the moment she swished across TV screens uttering the immortal phrase, 'Come on, girls, let's say it – because we're worth it!' in her first solo L'Oréal ad.

'I was so flattered when they asked me,' she confided to *Hello!* magazine. 'I thought, "They can't be serious!"'

CHERYL'S TATTOOS

★ Tribal pattern underneath her little finger on the side of her right hand.
★ Private design on her left bum cheek.
★ Butterfly combined with a tribal design in the small of her back.
★ 'Mrs C' on the back of her neck.
★ Barbed wire, rose and treble clef around the top of her right thigh.

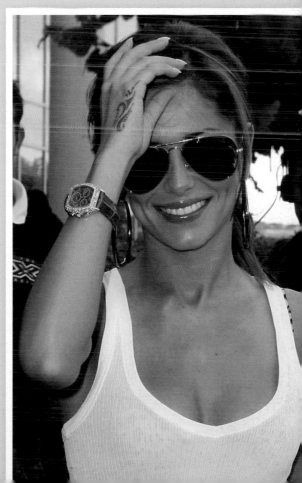

CHERYL'S HAIR:
A TIMELINE

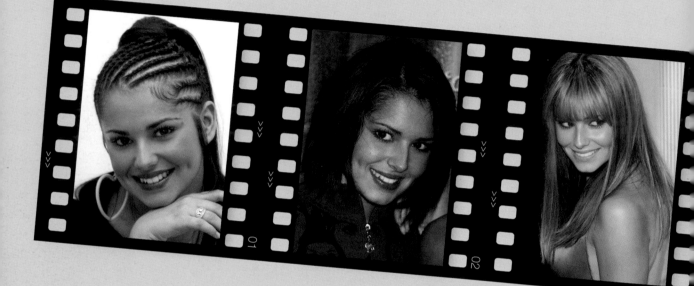

01 Cornrows

02 Bob with red chunks

03 Honey blonde with fringe

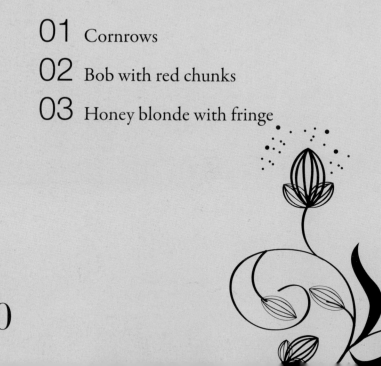

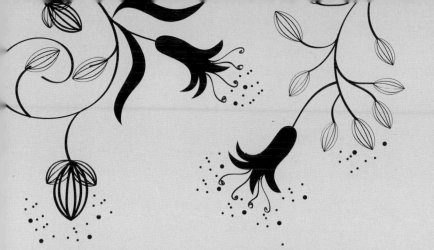

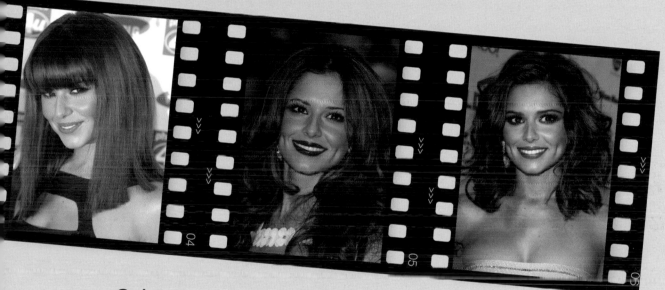

04 Brunette with fringe

05 Classic Cheryl – huge and brunette

06 Shoulder-length and wavy

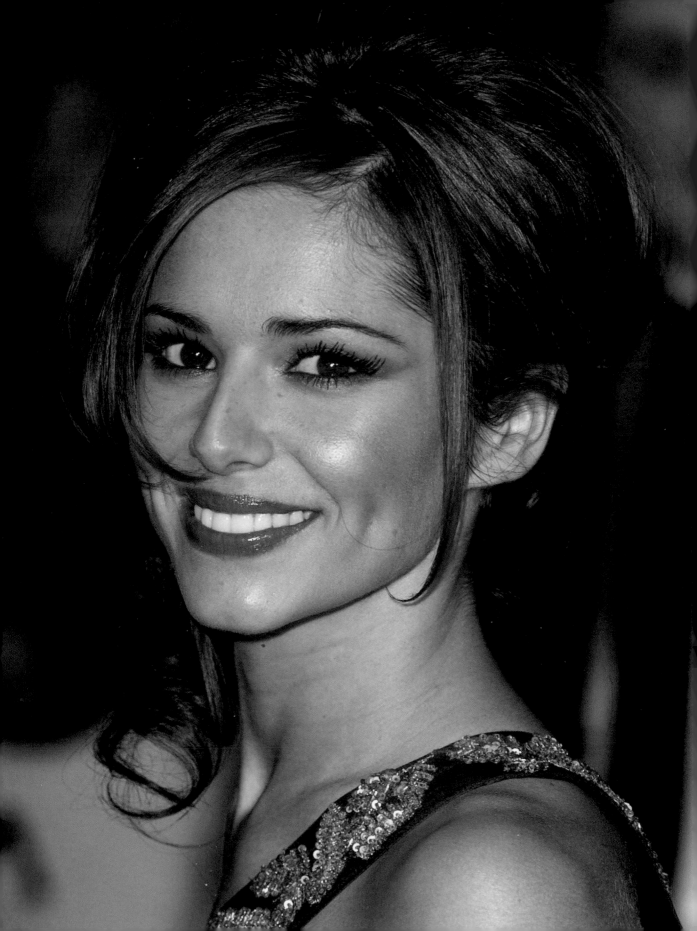

HAIR UP

Cheryl is most comfortable wearing her hair down, but as a girl who likes to play with different looks, there are certain times when she has been known to rock an up-do.

For red-carpet events and on *The X Factor*, she has experimented with neat, subtle beehives and a few cute and tidy 'do's – but is most keen on wearing it loosely piled up, with stray tendrils trailing around her face.

In recent years, she has been through the 'Cheryl style refinery', yet there are still touches of the urbanized teen who first hit the big time: the infamous 'Croydon facelift'-style scraped-back high ponytail resurfaced at her twenty-sixth birthday party. She also sometimes weaves skinny plaits or a couple of cornrows through her do to keep her feeling young and funky.

As a jewellery fan, Cheryl likes to accessorize her hair, too. She has alternated between delicately stranded Alice bands (which she also favours for a more casual look) and sparkling barrettes – and even on one occasion a jaunty kitty bow.

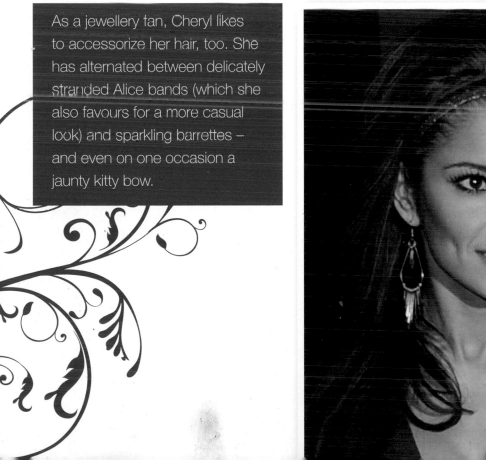

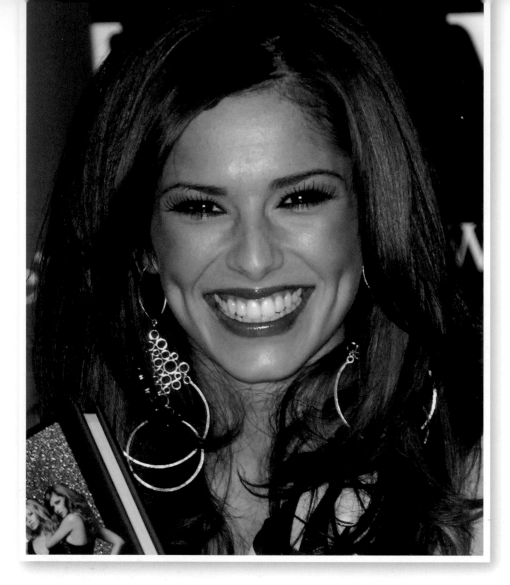

THE SMILE

If Cheryl's defining physical characteristic has become her hair, then her pearly whites definitely come in a close second.

Thanks to the warm smile that has encouraged many a young hopeful in the gruelling *X Factor* auditions, dazzled the photographers on the red carpet, and beamed modestly at the end of a successful performance, every molar has come in for inspection.

BRACE YOURSELF

Much has been made of the fact that Cheryl has altered her teeth since she first came into the public eye – but she hasn't come in for the stick that has been given her *X Factor* boss Simon Cowell for his Tipp-Ex white grin. Rather than change herself beyond all recognition, she has mainly worked with what she was given.

Back in 2005, she told the *News of the World*, 'On pictures I see this one tooth that I don't like and I always notice it.' So it's no surprise that four years later she revealed in *OK!* magazine, 'I actually wore a brace for two years – one of the Invisalign ones.'

Dr Hap Gill, from Smile Studio, believes that Cheryl's also had a few veneers, but in typical Cheryl style she hasn't overdone it and gone for a mouthful of porcelain.

Gill told the *Daily Star* he thought she had gone for more than just a brace, stating that in his opinion, 'Cheryl has had between six and eight veneers to give her a classic Hollywood smile.'

Invisalign braces have become hugely popular with many stars because they are so discreet and can be worn all the time, often only being noticed up close.

Oprah Winfrey, Heidi Klum and Katherine Heigl have also opted for Invisalign, where moulds of the teeth are taken and the soft clear plastic brace fitted; it is then changed every few weeks as the teeth move. It's expensive, costing around £2,000, but any dentist can make a referral for treatment.

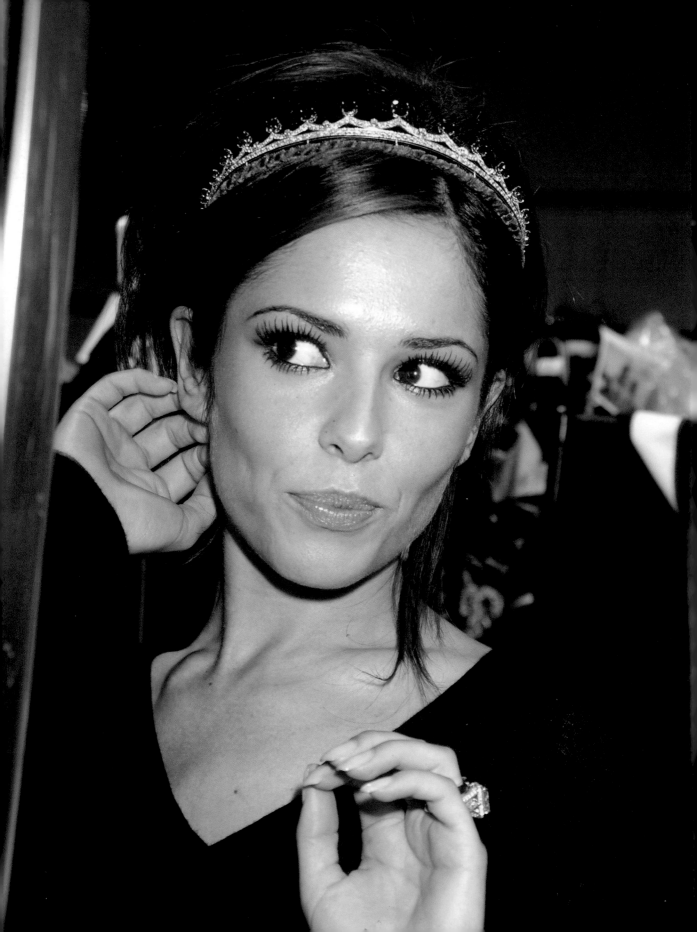

THE MAKE-UP

Always occasion-appropriate – whether her look is suitably OTT for the stage, striking for the TV cameras, or subtle during the day – Cheryl follows in the footsteps of stars from the golden age of Hollywood when it comes to her make-up.

For those who want to emulate her style, beauty expert Madeleine Crisp told the *Mirror*, 'Her signature look is very sexy and classic with simple smoky eyes, glossy skin and nude lips. She often frames her eyes with thick false eyelashes and mascara and defines them with eyeliner.'

'I prefer shopping for make-up than for clothes. I think it's exciting – all the new colours and things you can experiment with.'

Girls Aloud Style

Cheryl admits that perfume is one of her big weaknesses: she is always buying new fragrances and never wearing them. Two of her favourites are Hugo Boss Orange eau de toilette, and Viktor & Rolf Flowerbomb.

A HELPING HAND

For any professional event, Cheryl employs the expertise of her long-standing make-up artist Lisa Laudat, who has also worked with the rest of Girls Aloud, as well as Sophie Ellis-Bextor, Amy Winehouse and Corinne Bailey Rae.

It's natural that stars rely on trusted collaborators, and it goes beyond diva demands – when it's your job to look your best, you don't want to be standing in front of the cameras not feeling like yourself.

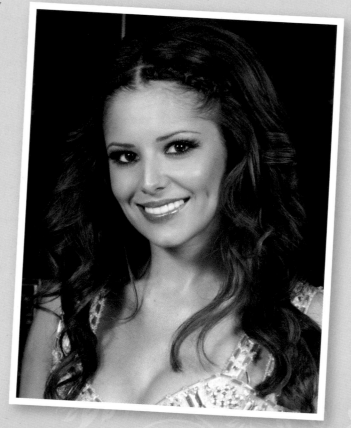

Cheryl once told *The Sun* that she often doesn't like the way her make-up is done on TV shows overseas because they make her look like she's in drag, explaining, 'They use different stuff and I end up all rosy cheeks and big black eyes!'

Away from the studio lights, for day-to-day Cheryl does her own make-up.

THE SECRET WEAPONS

Every woman has a handful of essential products in her make-up bag that form the foundations of her look – and Cheryl is no different.

Even before signing to cosmetics firm L'Oréal, she had always raved about their products, so it's no surprise that their Volume Shocking mascara and True Match roll-on foundation are two of her favourites.

Of the foundation, she said to *Glamour* online, 'It's just so quick. It's really clever. There's a lot of times when I'm running late, I'm just looking a bit rubbish because it's early, I haven't got time or I can't function enough to sit down and put my make-up on – so I find that fantastic. It's the simplicity.'

Although she is blessed with great skin, Cheryl believes in lending Mother Nature a little helping hand. Consequently, she always carries MAC face and body foundation in her make-up bag for her arms and legs, telling *Girls Aloud Style*, 'It's really light on your skin; it's like a second skin, almost, to make it all look one tone.'

And make-up artist Lisa Laudat revealed another tip to getting Cheryl's enviable glowing complexion. Speaking to *Grazia* online after one of Cheryl's *X Factor* appearances, Lisa said, 'I used the mineral foundation from Youngblood Cosmetics as it evens out her skin tone without smothering too much, leaving behind that radiance.'

Mineral make-up works with the wearer's skin – it doesn't block pores like a lot of make-up, and it also reflects light, leaving skin with a natural-looking glow.

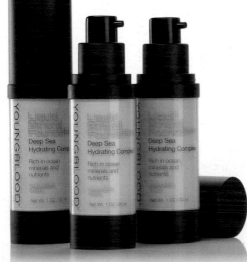

CHERYL'S MAKE-UP: A HOW-TO GUIDE

DEWY COMPLEXION Cheryl loves L'Oréal True Match foundation. For a really natural look, she advises mixing a little bit of foundation with moisturizer to create a gently tinted moisturizer.

LIGHT BLUSH She likes cream blusher because powder sits on the skin. To work out where to apply, she advises smiling and dabbing it onto the apples of the cheeks.

EYELINER She favours Shu Uemura, telling *Girls Aloud Style*, 'I only wear a little bit, but I use it quite a lot.'

Cheryl adds that if you want to wear liquid eyeliner, you should draw it on with pencil first and then paint the liquid over the top.

FALSE EYELASHES Apart from for work, Cheryl only wears false eyelashes on special occasions.

She likes the Shu Uemura range as they specialize in elaborate and theatrical designs, but for more traditional glamour, she and her bandmates helped to design a range of lashes for Eylure.

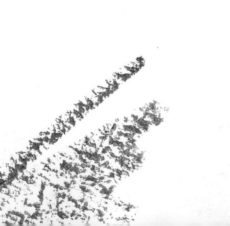
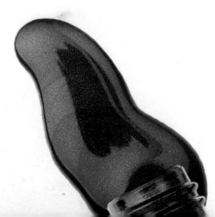

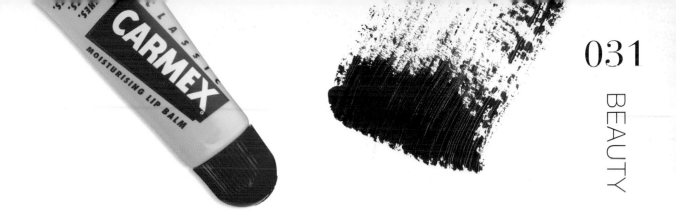

LIPS

She keeps her lips soft with Carmex lip balm and relies on L'Oréal for colour and shine. She tends to keep her lip shade subtle during the day, but often wears a pop of colour like red or fuchsia for TV or evenings.

She's the face of L'Oréal's Glam Shine reflection lip gloss, but insists she's always been a fan, telling *OK!* magazine, 'I've always worn Glam Shine because it's one of those lip glosses that doesn't stick. Sheer Cassis is my favourite because it works with my skin tone.'

MASCARA

L'Oréal Volume Shocking is Cheryl's mascara of choice. She told *Girls Aloud Style*, 'When I'm putting mascara on, I try to get every single eyelash, even the tiny little ones in the corner, because it makes you look like you've got a bigger eye.'

She puts it on the underside first and then a little bit on the top, and advises using lengthening mascara if you have short lashes, or thickening if you have long lashes.

Cheryl adds that you shouldn't keep mascara for too long: 'If it doesn't make that fresh popping sound when you take the wand out, then throw it away.'

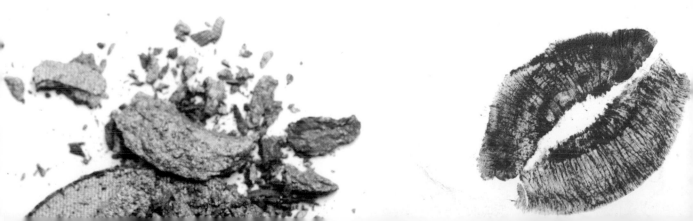

OFF-DUTY: ON CAMERA

While some grungier stars pride themselves on going bare-faced and low-key away from the red carpet and the film cameras, thankfully Cheryl is not one of them.

She believes in drawing a clear line between work life and private life when it comes to her make-up – but having grown up in the age of long-lens paparazzi, she knows she could get snapped at any moment and so ensures she always looks immaculate, even when she is officially 'off-duty'.

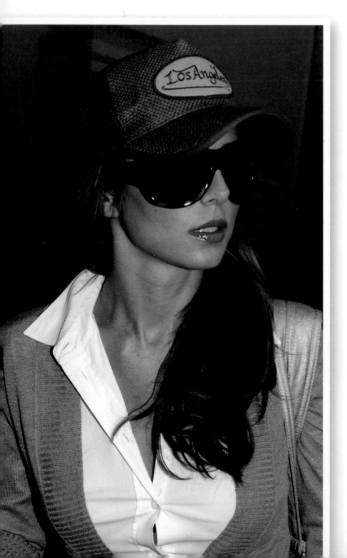

She has learnt from previous experience. It dates back to when she was once caught on camera going into a recording studio with no make-up on and spot cream dotted all over her face. She vowed there and then: never again! As she told *Sugar* magazine, 'From the moment I step outside my front door – even if it's just to go to the supermarket – I'm working.'

Her position is also a way of protecting herself. As she wrapped up an interview with *Elle* magazine, the journalist informed her that a group of paparazzi had gathered outside. So, the singer asked to borrow the interviewer's mascara for a quick touch-up, explaining, 'If they're gonna get a picture, I'm not going to let them get a bad one.'

'Exfoliating helps bad circulation and makes your skin softer, so I do it twice a week and I've really noticed the difference.' *Glamour* online

THE BEAUTY REGIME

While the lipstick, powder and paint are all very well to create that all-important showbiz face for the cameras, Cheryl realizes the importance of making sure you look after what you've got underneath. She said in an online chat, 'I always take my make-up off at night, no matter how tired I am, and I always moisturize my face.'

She uses a face cloth as she has a phobia of cotton wool, explaining in the Girls Aloud autobiography *Dreams That Glitter*, 'I never use it, not for taking my make up off or anything. Even when I get my nails done, they use tissues. Just the feel of it ... it squeaks. Urgh. I can't bear it.'

When she was growing up, the family home had a bath, but no shower, so Cheryl prefers baths, adding to *Glamour* online, 'Although I shower in the mornings, I prefer having a bath to exfoliate or shave my legs.'

Sticking with the L'Oréal range, she favours their Pure Zone Step 1 for her exfoliating needs.

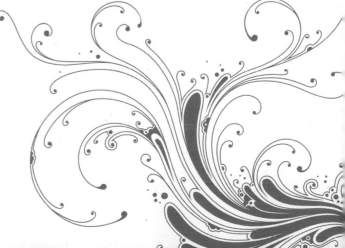

THE NAILS

Her nails are always manicured, but she usually favours a natural look with her nails left bare or enhanced with a simple French manicure. Occasionally, she favours darker colours like burgundy, purple or navy.

She has worn the eco-friendly LA brand Nubar, which is also popular with Eva Mendes, Rihanna and Scarlett Johansson, choosing the Navy Blue for an episode of *The X Factor*.

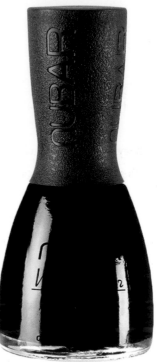

HAPPY TOES

Whenever Cheryl's spirits are in need of a boost, her quick fix is to paint her nails! She refers to digits with brightly painted nails as 'happy fingers' or 'happy toes', telling *Celebs on Sunday* magazine, 'You look at your toes a lot, don't you? So I call them my happy toes and painted them all bright shiny pink. Every time I look at my feet, I feel happy. It's a new discovery of mine. It makes you feel happier and it gives you a little surge.'

THE EYEBROWS

Cheryl prefers to pluck her own eyebrows rather than opt for celeb favourites such as waxing or threading.

Although she has revealed that even in recent years she plucked her brows far too thin and really regretted it, it hasn't stopped her tending to them herself. She told *Hello!* magazine, 'I always pluck my eyebrows when I get out of the shower because it's less painful, as I have such thick brows.'

EXTREME TREATMENTS

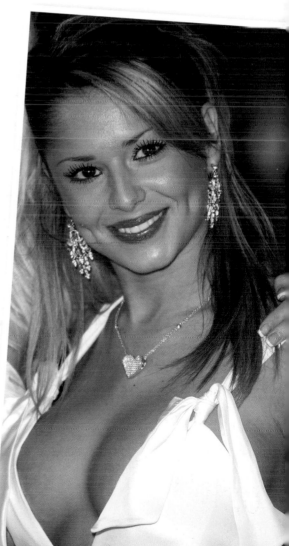

There have been suggestions Cheryl has gone under the knife for breast augmentation and under the needle for Botox, but she has vehemently denied both, adding to *Grazia*, 'In an ideal world, I'd have smaller boobs. I'm a 32D, which is ridiculous for my size, and boobs are hard to dress. I hate looking booby. You can look really cheap very quickly.'

And she stated in *Dreams That Glitter*, 'People don't even know the consequences of Botox yet; it hasn't been round long enough for people to know what's going to happen to your face in twenty years' time.'

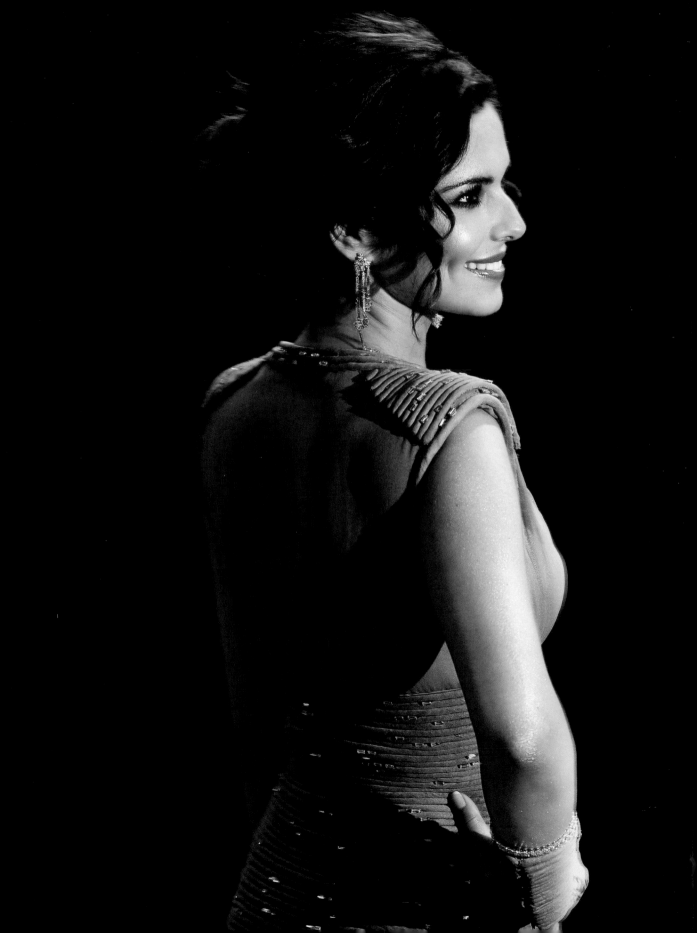

'People go on about the bump in my nose, but I don't mind. It's character.'

Dreams That Glitter

INDIVIDUALITY

While some women in the public eye, such as Katie Price and Heidi Montag, have made no secret of the fact they strive for perfection and will go through numerous extensive and painful operations where surgeons shave bones, suck fat, slice up and re-sew the ladies on their operating tables like Frankenstein's fembots, Cheryl is keen to stress that although it's OK to enhance what you've been given in a way that adds to rather than changes you, it's better to learn to accept physical imperfections.

'We're all individuals and the quirky things make a character,' she explained in *Dreams That Glitter*. 'You normally find it's the imperfections and insecurities that attract you to someone. I wouldn't mess around with my face ... in this industry, you come across a lot of "done" faces and you think, "Actually, she looked better before because she was unique."

'You can't make a doll, can you? You could make yourself perfect, but then you wouldn't be you.'

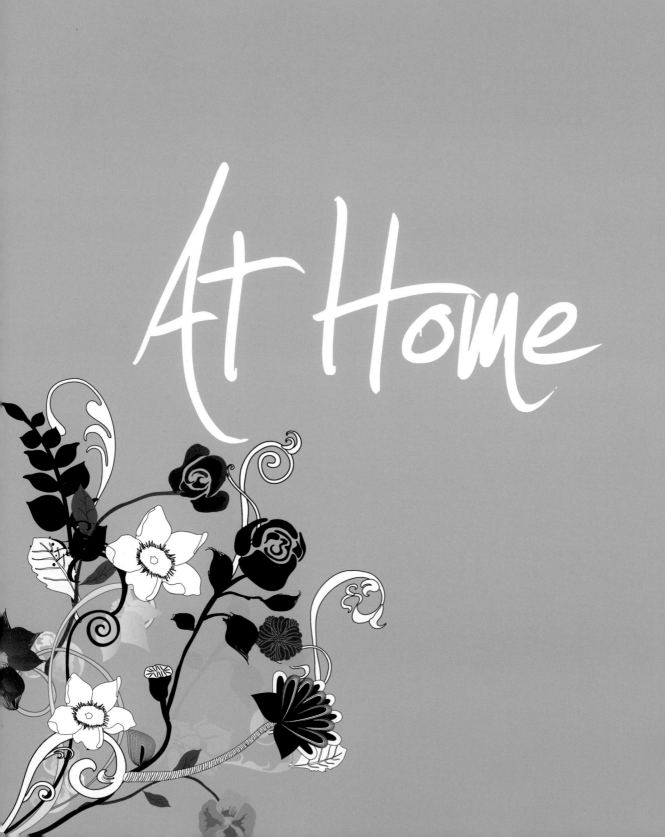

At Home

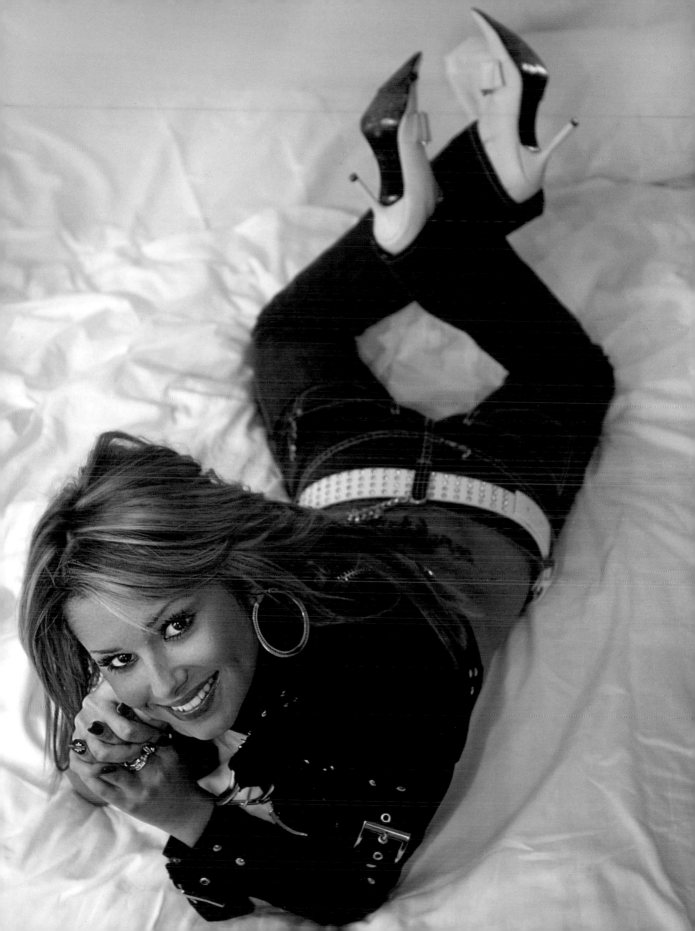

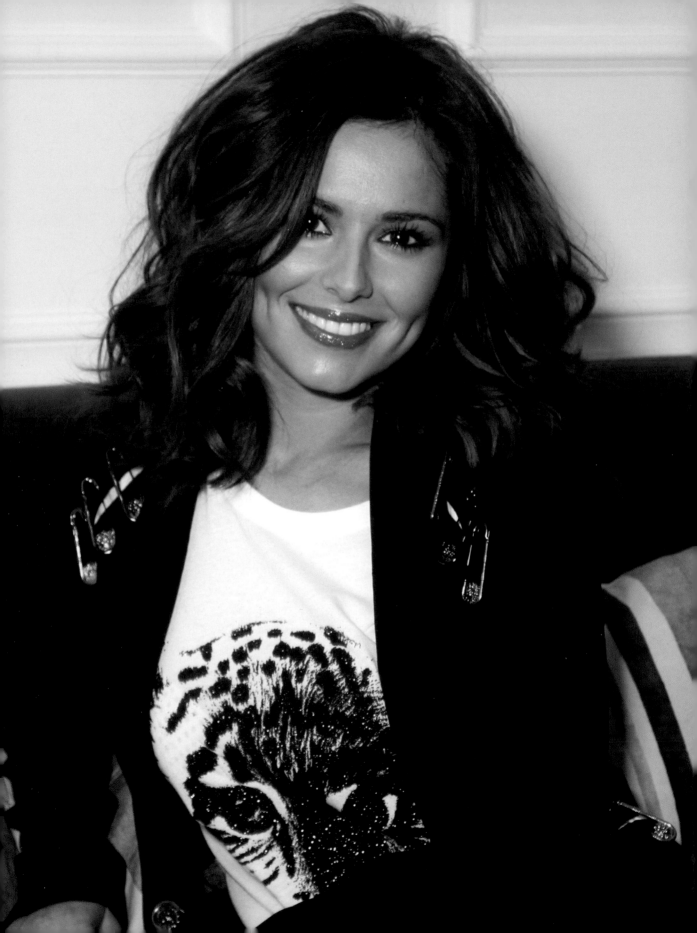

Cheryl: the provocative pop princess. Cheryl: the immaculate Saturday night TV star. Cheryl: the compassionate mentor. Cheryl: the fun-loving girlie girl. Wronged woman, style icon, national treasure, lads' mag pin-up … but who is she when she closes her front door behind her?

After spending so much time in the public eye, it's a Cheryl who incorporates all of these aspects when she is at home – yet home is also a place where she can be silly and vulnerable and scruffy and quiet.

'What I do love to do in my free time is watch the British soaps and spend time with my little dogs.' *OK!*

SIMPLE TASTES

It's been said that celebrities will always remain crystallized in time at the age at which they first became famous – and in some ways, despite the lacquer of stardom and years of experience in the entertainment industry, you can still see in Cheryl the nervous, emotional and hard-working nineteen-year-old who first emerged on *Popstars: The Rivals* in 2002.

And despite – or perhaps because of – the fact she has five-star hotels, free-flowing champagne and designer clothes all constantly within her grasp, her tastes are actually still very simple too.

'My perfect Sunday is at home watching the omnibus of the soaps, drinking a cup of English breakfast tea with sugar and milk, eating biscuits and snuggling my chihuahuas,' she told *OK!* magazine.

COUNTRY LIVING

When Cheryl and her bandmates first won a place in Girls Aloud, they were all put up in a north London luxury apartment complex, but ever since she gained financial independence, Cheryl has taken control of where she lives and has always opted for leafy countryside over living in the city.

She was just twenty-two when she bought her first home. While most people at that age would still be enjoying the bright lights and fast pace of a big city, Cheryl made it clear what her priorities were when she moved to suburban Hertfordshire.

She first got a taste of rural living when the ten *Popstars...* finalists shared a communal house in Surrey. Cheryl loved the area so much that it's where she has since returned to, currently living in Hurtmore House near Godalming.

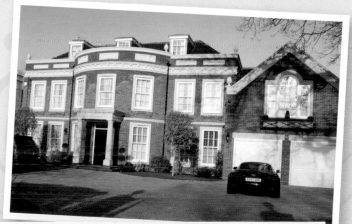

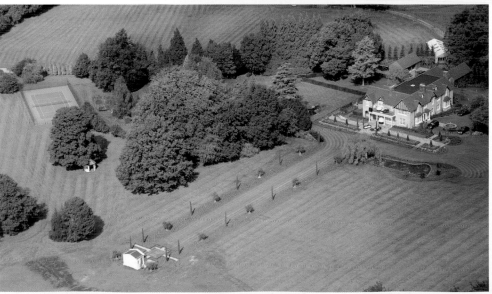

THROUGH THE KEYHOLE

When she first moved in at the beginning of 2009 – having purchased the Victorian property for £3.5 million – it was her absolute dream home.

It boasts nine bedrooms, and sprawling grounds with ponds dotted about. Deer roam through the acres of land, which is a real plus for Cheryl, as she is a devoted animal-lover.

Inside the house, the décor is high glamour all the way, with an indoor pool, a gym and a dressing room, which she described to *Vogue* as 'a big, bright pink Audrey Hepburn room', with black carpets, black chandeliers and silver, faux-snakeskin walls.

MOVING ON

In the light of Cheryl's divorce, however, Hurtmore House has ceased to be a happy home, and Cheryl is now considering her options. After she filed for divorce, a source close to her told *The Sun* newspaper, 'The house means nothing to her. Cheryl is giving the house to [Ashley].'

Cheryl may decide to set up home in LA. America has been a welcome retreat for the singer in recent months, and if her work in the US continues to go well, it could be the perfect base for her as her international career flourishes.

SCENT OF SUCCESS

A nice smell is really important to Cheryl; perfume is one of her weaknesses. She likes her home to smell fragrant too, telling *Glamour* online, 'I love scented candles – they're all gone within a couple of days! I like floral or appley, cinnamon smells.'

Cheryl even says she likes the smell of bleach – although she's not often the one using it to clean her home. She's confessed she doesn't do much housework and those close to her have always said she is very messy – her *X Factor* colleague Louis Walsh even revealed that her dressing room is a tip!

Thankfully, she has a cleaner at home, who comes once a week.

'I love scented candles. I like floral or appley, cinnamon smells.' *Glamour* online

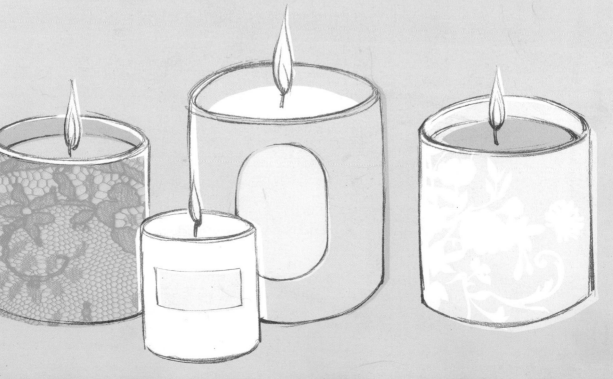

GUILTY PLEASURES

Like most people, Cheryl likes to get in from work, flop on the sofa and watch a bit of TV. It doesn't matter that her work takes her into stadiums and studios, she will still come home and get stuck into an episode of one of her favourite programmes – either *Coronation Street* or *EastEnders*, although she also loves reality TV and addictive US shows that she calls her 'guilty pleasures'.

In *Dreams That Glitter*, she confessed, 'When I get in at night, I have a shower, put my pyjamas on and watch TV – the soaps and trashy American shows I shouldn't really admit to, like *Maury* and *Ricki Lake*.' She also loves *The Hills* and told *OK!* magazine, '*The Hills* is the best programme ever.'

If she's not watching the box, Cheryl enjoys playing games on her Wii, and has revealed that one of her favourites is Sonic the Hedgehog.

GETTING PAMPERED

Despite having the skills of top beauty therapists at her perfectly manicured fingertips, Cheryl is actually not a big fan of spa treatments and has said that she prefers to relax by watching TV, playing with her dogs and cuddling up on the sofa in her pyjamas, rather than getting wrapped, scrubbed and pummelled.

As she employs the services of hair and make-up experts and manicurists to make her camera-ready, she views that process as more of a necessity for work, and therefore not a pampering treat. She told *Glamour* online, 'I'm not the sort of girl who enjoys being pampered. I can't get into massages – I can't relax.'

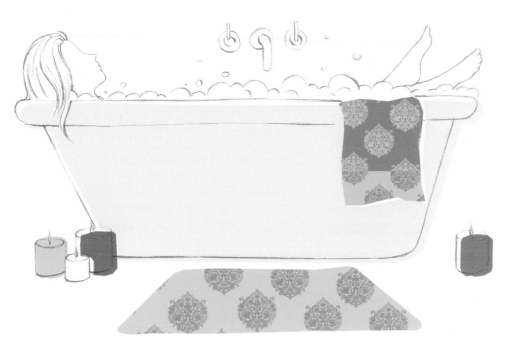

So even though she has visited hotels with some of the most luxurious spas in the world, she prefers the DIY approach, telling *The Sun*, 'I prefer to pamper myself just sitting in the bath.'

CHERYL'S 'RELAXING AT HOME' CHECKLIST

★ Pyjamas
★ Tea (milk, two sugars)
★ Biscuits (HobNobs)
★ Her chihuahuas (Buster and Coco)
★ *Coronation Street* and *EastEnders* omnibuses

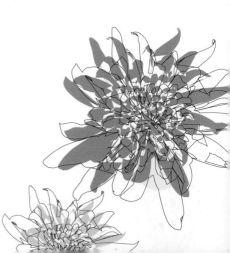

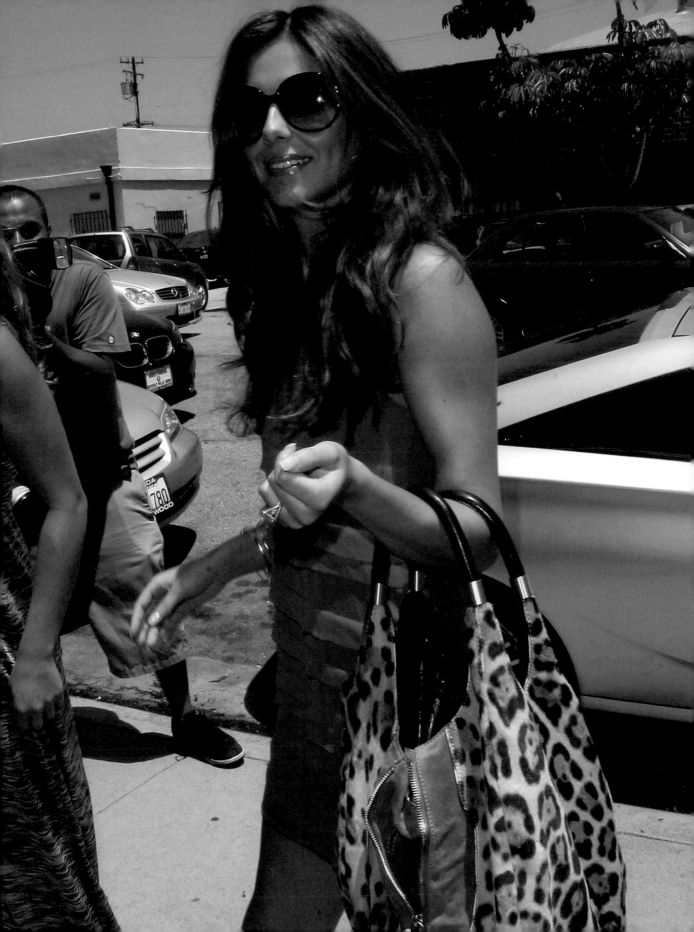

PYJAMAS AND FLUFFY SLIPPERS

Cheryl always looks so immaculate when she steps out into the public eye that it's easy to imagine her dressed the same at home – striding around her country estate in monster heels with an outsized bag over the crook of her arm.

But that vision couldn't be further from the truth. After being winched into stilettos, lashed into corsets and squeezed into skintight outfits for work, when she's at home, Cheryl likes to slob out in tracksuits, pyjamas and fluffy slippers, telling *Vogue*, 'I've got an obsession with snuggly pyjamas. Can you believe Kimberley gave me a box from Victoria's Secret with twenty pairs?'

HER 'BABIES'

Cheryl's home life would not be complete without two very special creatures. She has said that she trusts only her mother and her dogs – but that doesn't come close to describing just how much she adores her beloved chihuahuas Buster and Coco.

Buster joined her family first, back in 2005: a white-and-sandy-coloured puppy, who, Cheryl told *The Sun*, has a penchant for burying her knickers in the garden! He was soon followed by a second chihuahua called Coco, who is black and fawn.

'I don't trust anybody except my mother and my dogs … it's scary that you can love a small, hairy thing so much.' *The Times*

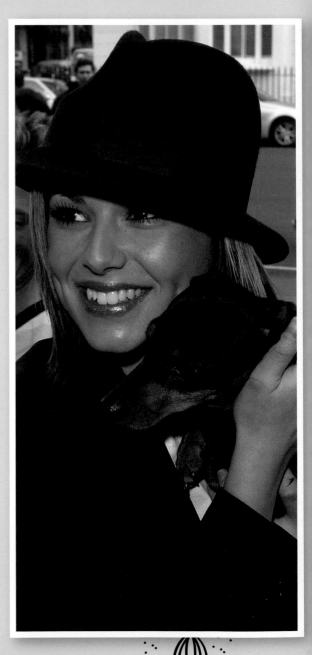

A DOG'S LIFE

Cheryl later told *The Times*, 'Buster is very loving. He needs to be cuddled constantly and wants to be stroked. Coco used to be schizophrenic and paranoid, but she's really changed. I drummed it into her you will be loved, you will enjoy cuddles and now she follows me all over the house. She's my little baby.'

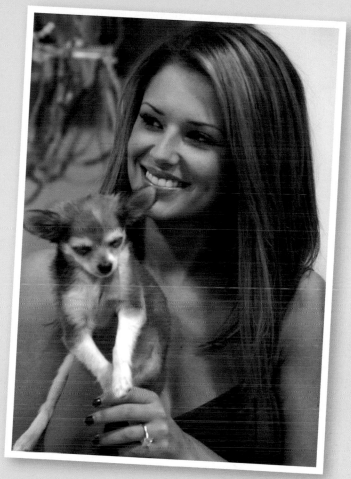

The little babies unfortunately have little accidents sometimes. Cheryl's ex-husband Ashley revealed in his autobiography *My Defence* that the dogs would occasionally mess on the floor. Once, Cheryl stood in it and had to hop to the bathroom – it's not all glamour in Cheryl's world!

Cheryl has bonded with Simon Cowell over their mutual love of dogs, as he has dogs of his own. The duo are often accompanied to the *X Factor* studios by their pets.

TEA AND SYMPATHY

One of Cheryl's absolute favourite things to do at home is put the kettle on. She truly is a girl of simple tastes, and explained almost apologetically on the TV show *Girls Aloud: Home Truths*, 'I love my cups of tea – I'm terrible for cups of tea!'

Later, on *Cheryl Cole's Night In*, she confided to Holly Willoughby that there was 'nothing better than watching a soap with a cup of tea and a HobNob'.

This passion is not a new one. Cheryl has revealed that before she found fame, she shared a flat with her boyfriend and all they had apart from a bed was a cup, a kettle, teabags, sugar and UHT (they didn't even have a fridge).

The singer is always keen to spread her love of a good cuppa. During her engagement shoot with *OK!*, she fussed round the magazine's team, making sure they were being looked after. 'She insisted on plying our crew with endless cups of tea,' the mag reported. 'She has definitely got a nurturing nature.'

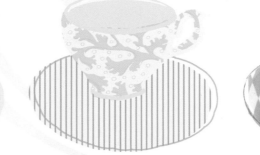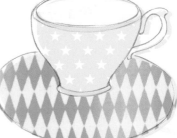

'I love my cups of tea – I'm terrible for cups of tea!'

Girls Aloud: Home Truths

HAPPY HOSTESS

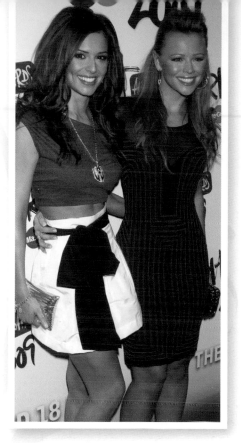

This nurturing nature makes for the perfect hostess, but Cheryl has confessed she's not good in the kitchen, commenting in *Dreams That Glitter*, 'I find cooking really therapeutic, but I'm not great at it. I'm learning.'

However, her lack of culinary talent doesn't stop her trying. For Ashley's birthday one year she hosted a kids' tea party for him, with buffet food like vol-au-vents and sausage rolls.

She also likes hosting for her pals and Kimberley Walsh revealed to *OK!* magazine: 'Cheryl likes having people round ... Just before Christmas I went round to hers and she'd done mulled wine and cheese and crackers and it was really nice. We hadn't seen each other for a while because she'd been busy, so we just sat down and started talking and didn't move from that spot!'

HER BELIEFS

Although Cheryl is primarily an entertainer, she is frequently asked for her views on a multitude of subjects in interviews – and her revelations make for thought-provoking reading, giving insight into her private philosophies, beliefs and opinions – and to how she might be as a dinner-party guest!

She's a complete mixture of common-sense street smarts, and girlie leap-of-faith whimsy, with opinions on everything from politics to astrology.

POLITICS

She told the *New Statesman*, 'Politicians know we get listened to by more young fans than they do. That's why David Cameron said he fancied me. Politicians should stop trying to be cool and get on with running the country.

'There should be adverts in the breaks during *Coronation Street* spelling it out in bullet points: This is what the Conservatives stand for. This is what Labour stands for.'

She added to *Q* magazine, 'We've always been Labour in our family, it just feels wrong not to be.'

FINANCIAL INDEPENDENCE

Throughout her relationship with Ashley, Cheryl was adamant about not being seen as a WAG – because of the negative connotations that come with the tag, concerning living off your husband's money and having none of your own ambitions.

She told *The Sun* in April 2006, 'I have my own credit cards. I would die of embarrassment if I had to resort to taking my

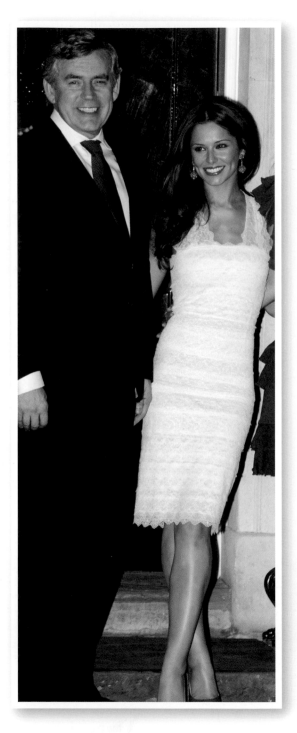

boyfriend's cards. When I met Ashley, I was already earning my own money and doing my own thing.'

Today, Cheryl's personal wealth is estimated at £10 million.

LIFE PHILOSOPHY
Cheryl has taken some hard knocks in life. Yet her overwhelming philosophy in life is to keep battling on against all the odds. Shortly before she began divorce proceedings against Ashley, she said on a Norwegian TV show, 'Sometimes things get tough, but you've just got to fight on. What are you going to do? Give up, curl into a ball or are you going to keep fighting on? My message is fight on. You can't give up and lie down. You've got to keep going.'

GHOSTS
When Cheryl appeared with her bandmates on the one-off TV show *Ghost-Hunting with Girls Aloud*, she spoke of her belief in ghosts and talked about orbs flying past her face and her hand being stroked by a spirit.

PSYCHICS
Cheryl consulted a psychic before she started going out with Ashley – and it was reported that she saw another one after they split up.

'I am like my star sign, cancer. I'm like a crab, hard on the outside and soft on the inside.' *OK!*

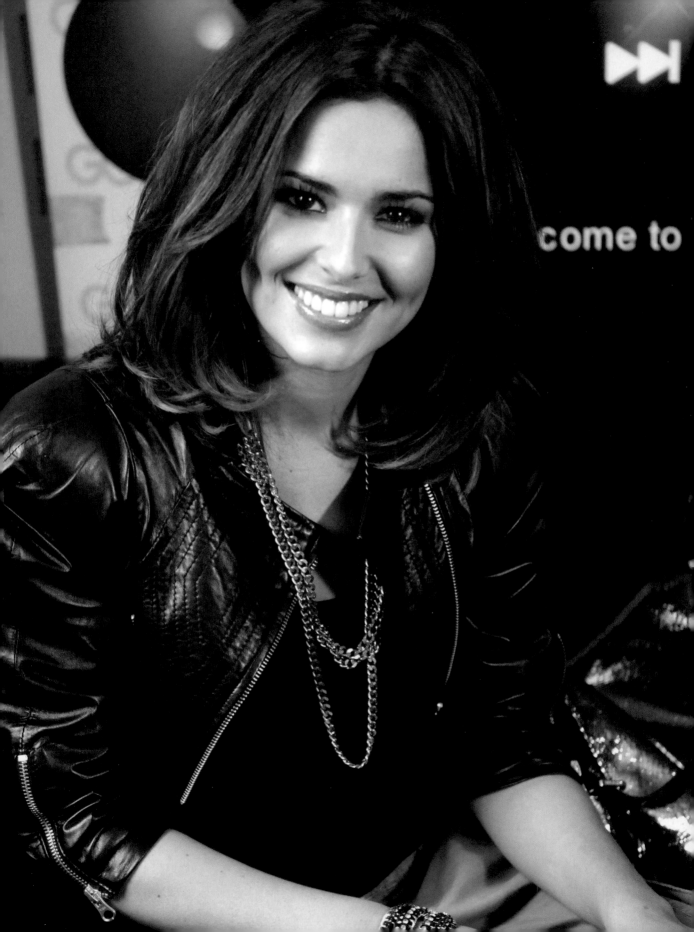

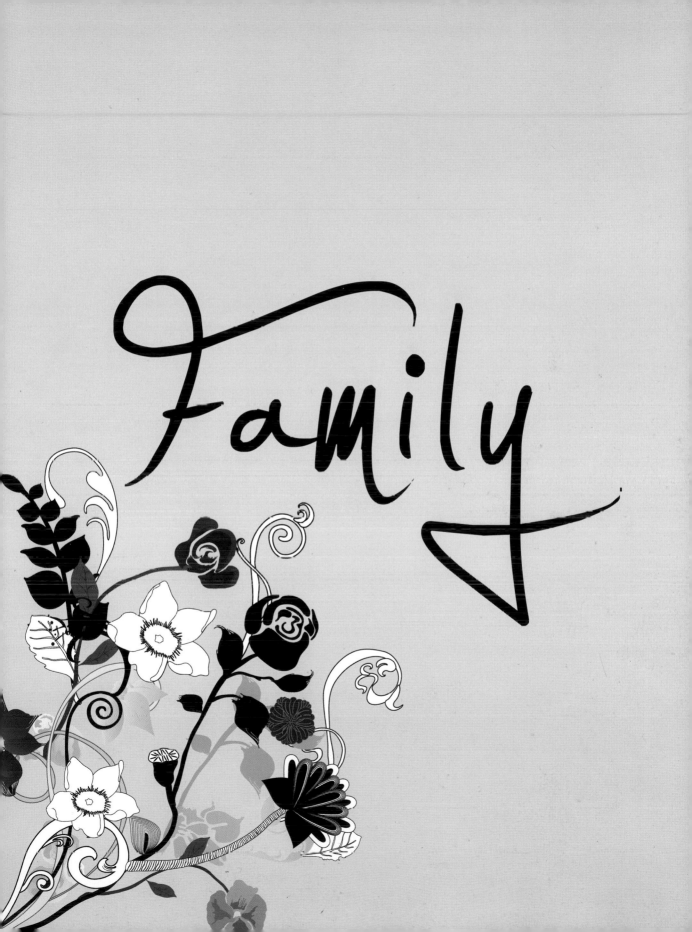

If music is the lifeblood that flows through Cheryl's veins, then her family are the heart that keeps her going. They are a big part of the person she is today.

Cheryl is a working-class girl from a very close family. They are one of the most important aspects of her life, especially her parents.

She still fights, cries and laughs with them, having learned the importance of loyalty, hard work and unconditional love from them while growing up.

She also has a host of siblings and – as you'd expect – is a dedicated sister to them all.

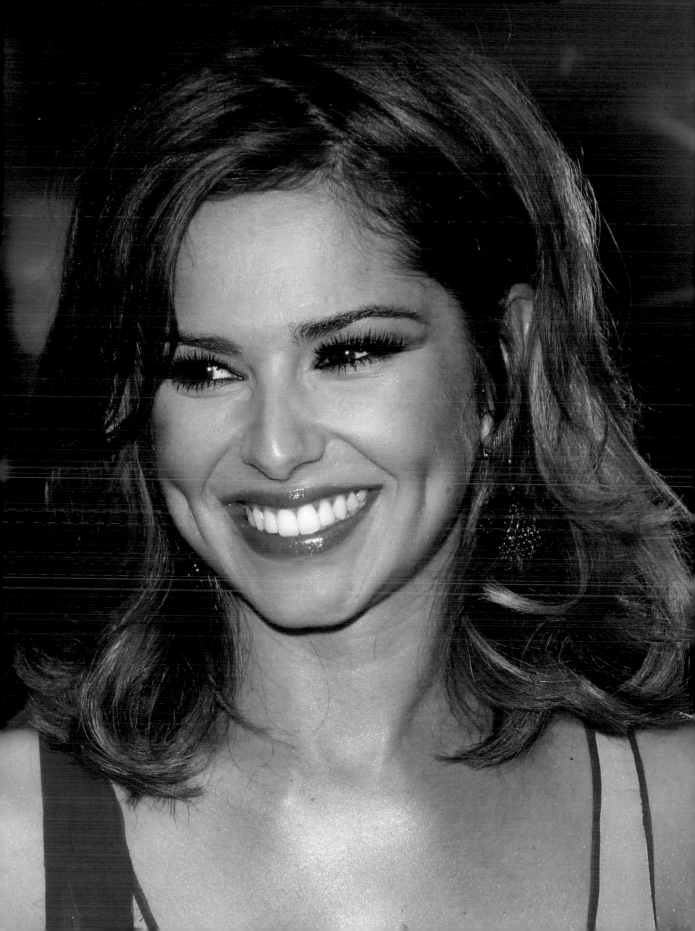

FAMILY AFFAIR

Cheryl says she has inherited qualities from both her parents and is still devoted to each of them. The singer has made no secret of the fact she's very emotional and says that her whole family are the same way.

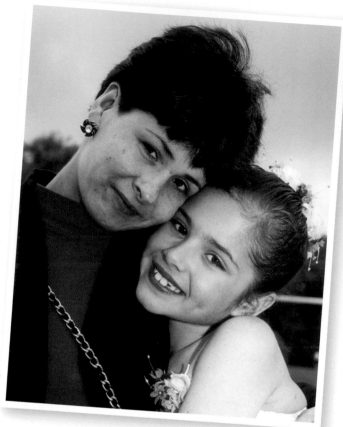

She is extremely close to her mum – seeing her as a sister or a friend as well as a mother – and the pair share many similarities, both physically and in terms of both being no-nonsense, family-oriented women.

Cheryl's also always had her father's stoic support, while her siblings are a huge part of her life too. She learned how to look after herself from her two older brothers, shared girlie secrets with her older sister, and is still very protective of her little brother.

Cheryl is also very close to the whole extended family, which includes a sprawling mass of Callaghans, Leightons, Bakers and Tweedys. Cheryl's parents split when she was eleven and her dad remarried, giving her a stepmother and assorted stepsiblings.

'MAM'

> **'Mam never really experienced the nice things in life, so now I like to spoil her.'** *Dreams That Glitter*

Despite being just a whisper over five foot in her stocking feet, Cheryl's mother Joan Callaghan is a formidable woman. With five kids to raise on very little money, life was frequently tough for Joan, but she is used to getting on with things and not making a fuss.

While she drove her youngest daughter to dance classes and made her costumes, encouraging her in her ambitions and being extremely proud of Cheryl for all that she has achieved, Joan is a grounded woman who will never let the celebrity lifestyle go to her daughter's head ... although that doesn't stop her from sampling its advantages.

The fun-loving pair often party together. Cheryl revealed to *The Sun*, 'Mum's a bigger clubber than me. She drags me onto the dance floor and doesn't stop moving.' She added to the *Mirror*, 'We get dressed up and have a right laugh.'

ROLE REVERSAL

Cheryl has said that there is a degree of role reversal between the two: her mum comes to her for advice and Cheryl told the *Mirror*, 'My mum is more like a friend. I can talk to her about anything.'

But Joan is a mother figure too, and a pillar of strength to her youngest daughter. When Cheryl's court case came up, back in 2003, her mother moved down south to stay with her for the week. Cheryl told *The Sun*, 'I couldn't have coped without her. She was my rock.'

Although Joan stays with Cheryl a lot in her Surrey home, she doesn't live with her daughter full-time as is frequently reported.

Cheryl's roots and where she comes from are really important to her. In the early days of Girls Aloud, she chose to support a cancer charity because her nanna, whom she 'loved to bits', died from breast cancer.

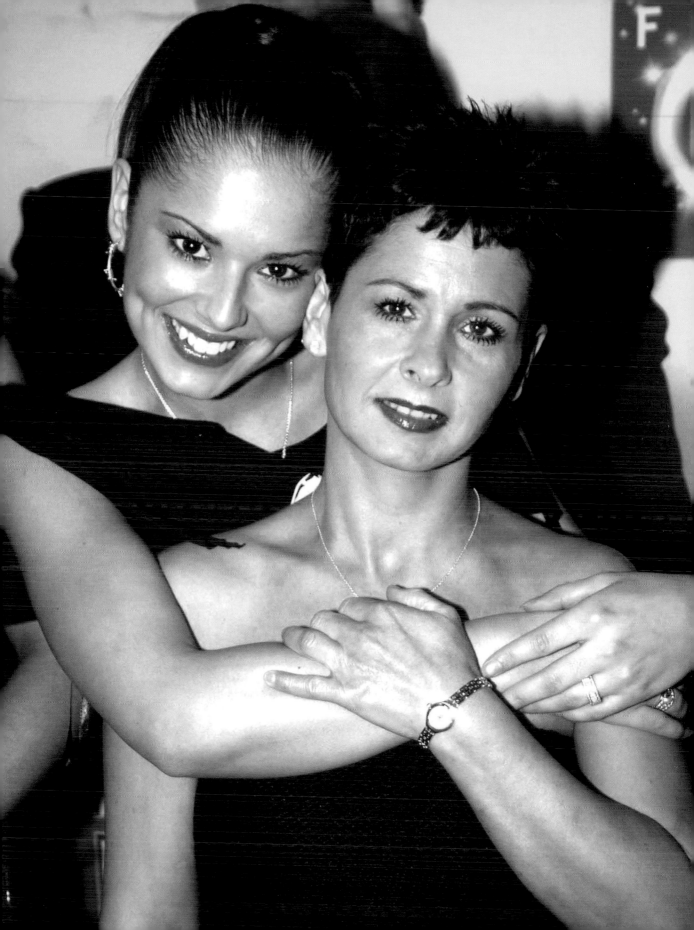

DAD

Cheryl is also very close to her dad Garry Tweedy. She clearly inherited her emotional nature from him, telling *The Times*, 'Sometimes he gets watery eyes just from talking about it [what Cheryl has achieved] and says, "I could burst with pride."'

Cheryl is full of praise for her father, appreciating his 'lovely nature'. As she continued to *The Times*, 'My dad met my mum when he was seventeen and she was twenty-one and she already had three kids. Amazing that he took that on.'

She gave him a special thank you in the sleeve notes for her album *3 Words*, saying, 'Dad – thanks for keeping it real. You remind me of my dream and that's what I am living no matter how hard it sometimes gets. Thank you for being there for me. I know how proud you are and I love u.'

For his part, it's obvious that Garry absolutely dotes on his daughter. As was later reported by *OK!* magazine, he struggled with his emotions on her wedding day, and said in his speech, 'When Cheryl was born, I thought I was handed an angel. It was the proudest day of my life. She's independent, smart and stunning – perfect in every way.'

'I couldn't ask for a better daughter.' Garry Tweedy, *OK!*

SIBLINGS

Growing up, Cheryl had three brothers and one sister: Joseph (seven years older), Gillian (four years older), Andrew (two years older) and Garry (two years younger). As with most families, she has had her differences with her siblings over the years, but they have always been there for each other – and remain so to this day.

When Cheryl got married in 2006, Gillian was her maid of honour – and Cheryl was there for her big sister when she gave birth to son Kedric in November 2008. Andrew told the *Mirror*, 'As soon as Gillian went into labour, Cheryl drove up from London.'

Though Cheryl discovered at the age of eleven that her eldest three siblings were actually half-siblings, it made no difference to her: they were still her blood and they had been there alongside her – fighting, loving each other and growing up under the same roof – her whole life.

Now that Cheryl's siblings have families of their own, 'Auntie Cheryl' dotes on her numerous young nieces and nephews, who bring out the maternal instinct she's had from a very young age.

Cheryl's start in showbiz was a family affair. She and little brother Garry used to team up as a modelling double act when they were kids, starring in adverts for local companies.

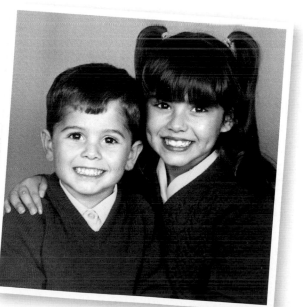

OH, BROTHER

Of all Cheryl's siblings, her brother Andrew has been the most troubled, and the biggest source of worry and upset to the family. Cheryl's relationship with him gives real insight into the tenacity of her emotions and her tendency always to see the best in people.

Andrew – who has been addicted to glue and alcohol since he was a teenager and who has been in court over fifty times, serving two jail sentences – is very much a product of his environment. Cheryl and her other siblings managed to escape the grasp of addiction and crime – but it's unsurprising that not *all* of her family were so fortunate.

For those who undermine what Cheryl has achieved, there's probably very little appreciation of the realities of what it's like to grow up with no money in an extremely rough area. It's those formidable early years that shaped her and made her the woman she is today.

Cheryl's family nickname is 'Chez'.

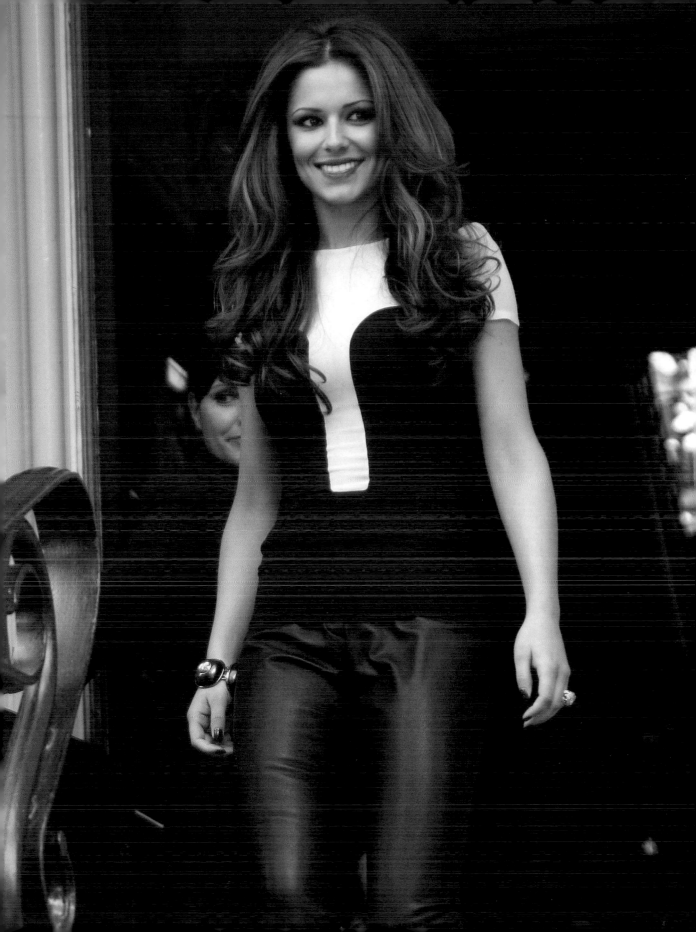

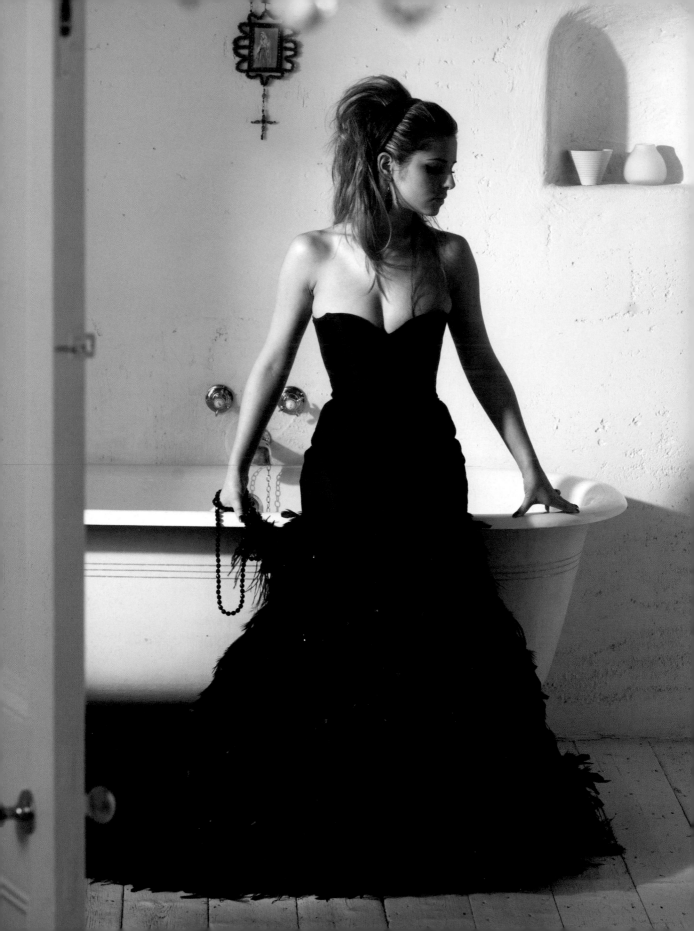

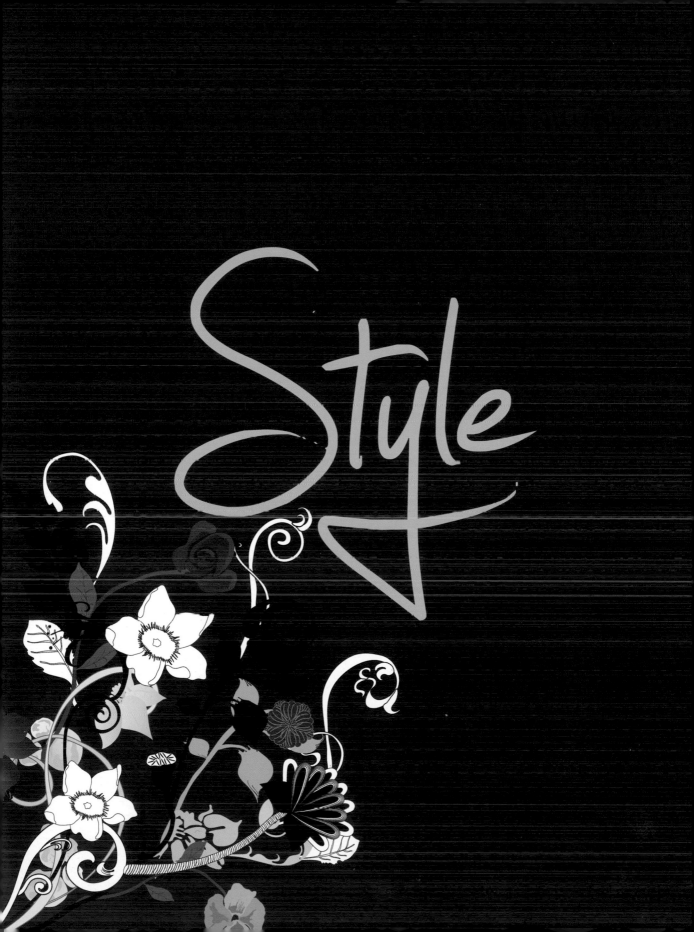

Cheryl has swiftly become one of the most stylish young women around. There are as many designers scrambling to clothe her as there are magazines desperate to have her grace their cover, and girls and women all over the world strive to emulate her look.

Glamour magazine editor Jo Elvin says, 'Cheryl Cole has become everyone's style crush. She's ridiculously gorgeous, beautifully groomed and always glossy, glossy, glossy.'

To cement this reputation, as the noughties – the decade in which Cheryl found fame – drew to a close, she was voted best-dressed woman by both *Tatler* and *Glamour* magazines and appeared on the cover of *Vogue*.

'I don't wear something just because someone is running down the catwalk in it.' *Elle*

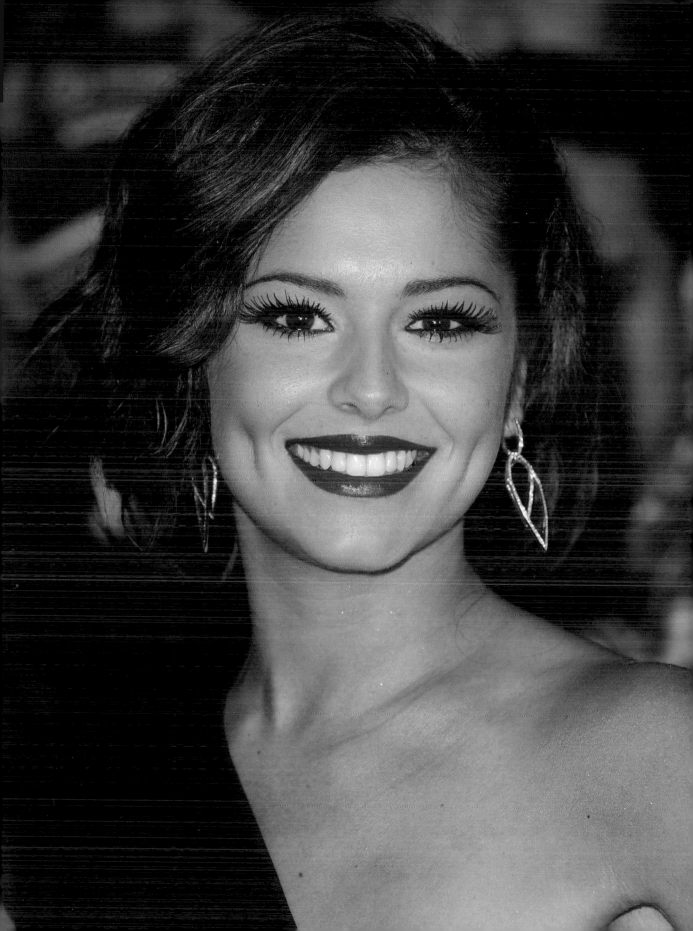

THE EARLY YEARS

The fashionista has certainly come a long way from the young girl who would have to borrow money if she wanted to afford something from River Island or Benetton, and who was teased by a local bully for wearing second-hand clothes.

Cheryl opened her heart to *Vogue* about those childhood experiences, saying, 'She would give [the hand-me-downs] to me herself when she was finished with them and then laugh when she'd see me clunking down the street in shoes stuffed with tissue paper because they were always too big.'

FIRST STEPS

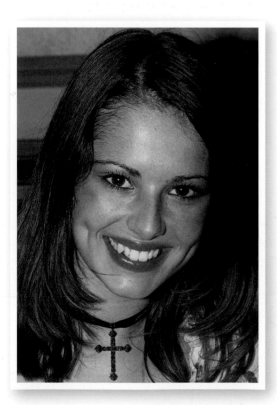

Cheryl the style icon emerged from inauspicious beginnings: in a floral chintzy top, low-rider jeans and with a cross hung on a piece of ribbon around her neck – her outfit for her first *Popstars: The Rivals* audition.

She told *Dreams That Glitter*, 'I'd bought a new outfit in Newcastle thinking I looked fine, but when I look back now, I don't know what I was thinking.'

As one-fifth of Girls Aloud, for many years she was lost in an explosion of candy-coloured crop tops and rolled-up combat trousers teamed with heels, while in her down time she would escape the razzamatazz in trucker caps and hoodies.

BIRTH OF A STYLE ICON

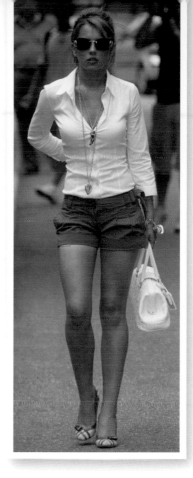

Perhaps the first inkling of Cheryl as fashionista came at the 2006 World Cup where, as the stadium floodlights were trained on the players, the flashbulbs of the world's press were firmly focused on the wives and girlfriends, and their style choices as they supported their menfolk from the sidelines and socialized together in the evenings.

While the other WAGs came in for some negative press, Cheryl and Victoria Beckham neatly sidestepped the main gaggle in mix 'n' match form-fitting dresses, sexy shorts, tumbling curly hair extensions, quirky pendants and fitted waistcoats.

Cheryl told the *Daily Star* at the time, 'Victoria is the most stylish. She always looks amazing to me. I love her Rock and Republic jeans, too. She gave me a pair when she first started designing them and I've bought loads more since then. They're expensive but, believe me, they're worth it.'

BRIDAL BOMBSHELL

When Cheryl wed in summer 2006, the event secured her blossoming fashion reputation.

For her big day, she opted for a figure-hugging ivory duchesse satin Roberto Cavalli gown, stitched with sequins, beads and diamante, which was scrutinized along with her choice of accessories and jewels.

The bride told *OK!* magazine, 'There's been loads of speculation that it was Victoria who put me in touch with Roberto Cavalli, but it was actually nothing to do with her. We just both love that designer. I looked through some of the designs Roberto had sketched and it turned out my favourite was his as well.'

While some people were perhaps expecting an overblown sugary confection of a dress teamed with a waterfall of diamonds, Cheryl received praise for keeping her styling simple and age-appropriate, with an understated yellow-and-white diamond Garrard tiara, and plain diamond studs in her ears. Although she did up the bling with her 8-carat yellow diamond heart wedding ring …

A STAR IS BORN

In spring 2009, Cheryl raised the style stakes to the max when she was invited to appear on the cover of *Vogue*. Satisfyingly, 'her' edition garnered the magazine's best-ever circulation for that month.

Indeed, *Vogue* editor Alexandra Shulman said, 'Cheryl Cole is the love object of the moment. Her winning appeal as an *X Factor* judge has catapulted her out of predictable WAG-dom to sitting rooms and the front pages of the national press.'

'Cheryl Cole is the love object of the moment.'

Alexandra Shulman, editor of *Vogue*

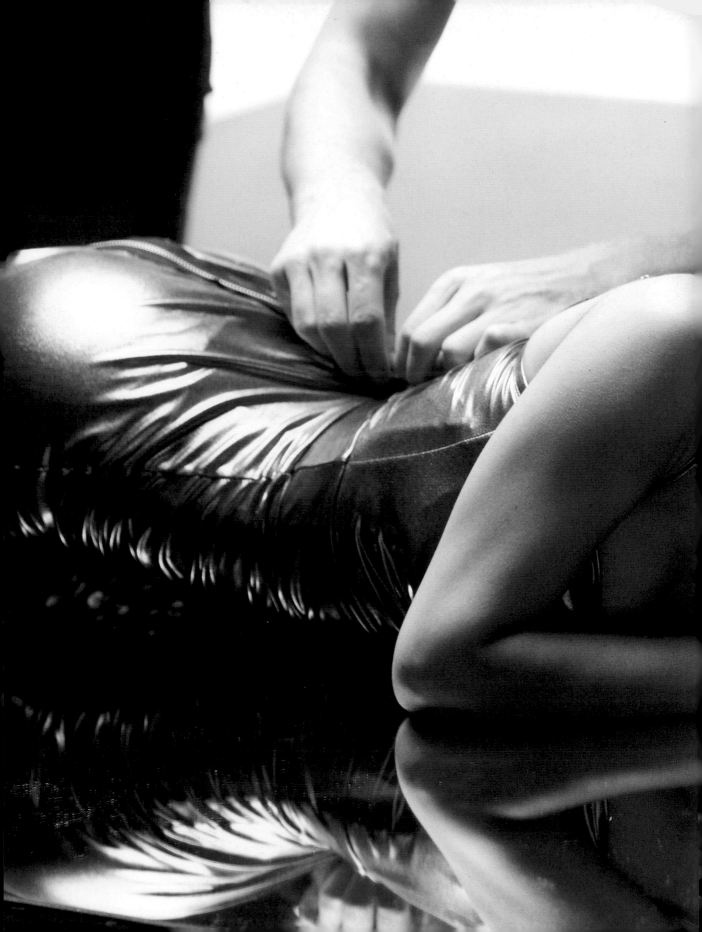

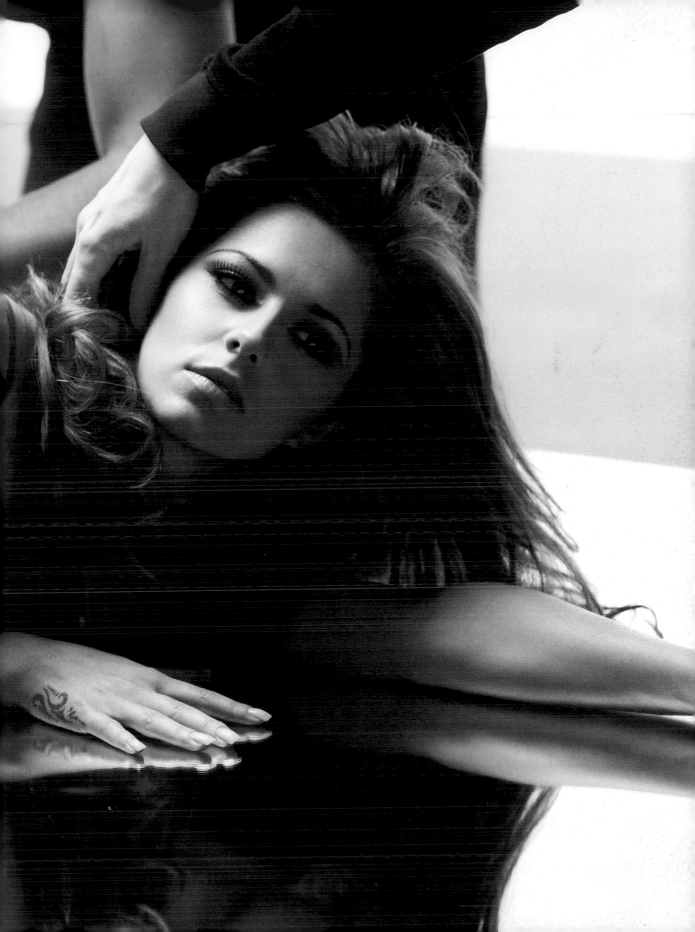

THE *VOGUE* EXPERIENCE

Cheryl's *Vogue* shoot was by no means a flawless event. It was remarked by the magazine that, even though the star wore designer labels – for the interview she teamed a cream-and-black Sonia Rykiel blouse with a puffball mini by Vanessa Bruno – she had nicks in her tights, you could see her hair extensions from the back, and her nails were unfiled.

These details did not go unnoticed by the notoriously unforgiving style bible, but they were all the more reason for the rest of the world to love her. These very human touches were also signs that, at that stage, Cheryl was still growing into her stratospheric celebrity – and her womanhood – at the age of twenty-five.

COMING OF AGE

If Cheryl's stellar style success were to be attributed to just one thing, it would have to be her role as judge on *The X Factor*.

Cheryl undoubtedly took the job because of her passion for music and her desire to help the next generation, but the perhaps unexpected upside was that she became a bona fide style star, raising the fashion stakes week after week with an enviable array of glamorous outfits.

Come 2009, and *GMTV* fashion presenter Mark Heyes told the *Mirror*, 'The X Factor has cemented Cheryl as a fashion icon.'

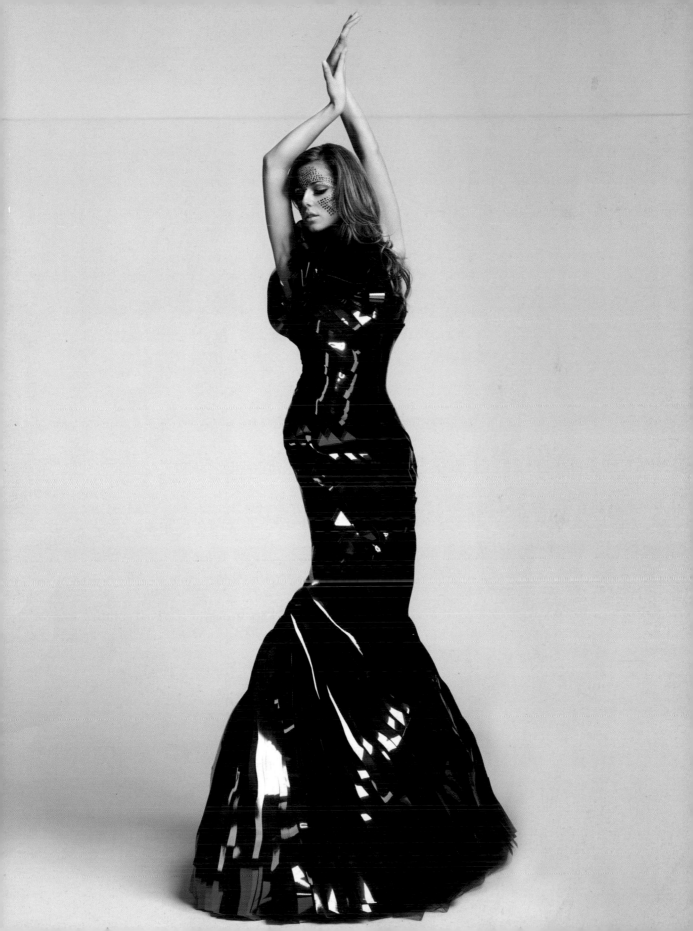

RED CARPET FABULOUS

Cheryl is now well used to putting on a show on the red carpet. She and her bandmates have evolved from sweet girls playing dress-up in floor-length gowns that seemed to swamp them at the *Love Actually* premiere to fully-fledged fashionistas, wowing the crowds at the BRIT Awards 2009, where they picked up their first BRIT: Best Single for 'The Promise'.

While the band put on a united front at the event in perfectly contrasted neutral tones, it was Cheryl who was singled out in the press the following day – for her bright white A-line minidress with appliqué flowers by up-and-coming designer Georges Chakra, teamed with silver double-strap Jimmy Choos and a slick of red lipstick.

Later, at one of her first solo appearances on the red carpet of a music event, she showed she was also capable of doing it alone. At the DLD Starnight awards ceremony in Germany in 2010, she was there to perform her single '3 Words', but also worked a nude Hervé Léger bandage dress for her strut down the red carpet – proving just how far she's come from the girl who admitted she used to pronounce the designer 'Harvey Ledger' ...

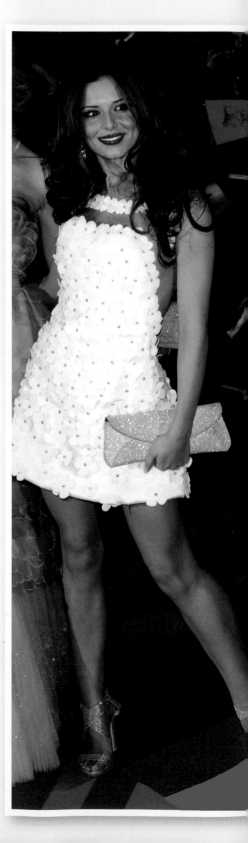

DAYWEAR

As well as learning how to work the red carpet, Cheryl has spent the past few years perfecting her daytime look.

Naturally, she has a great track record for getting it right, whether she is wearing a white lace Alexander McQueen bandage dress (with orange coral Kenneth Jay Lane earrings) for a post-Kilimanjaro trip to Downing Street, or strolling through an airport in leather leggings and a funky tank top.

For *The X Factor* auditions in her second series, she opted for all-out glamour, pouring herself into skinny jeans, cleavage-popping tops and killer heels; while for recording sessions for her debut solo album in LA, her wardrobe reflected the Californian sunshine, as she stepped out in a succession of cute, brightly coloured outfits, such as an aqua-and-white Alice + Olivia tunic, accessorized with a Vivienne Westwood teddy pendant.

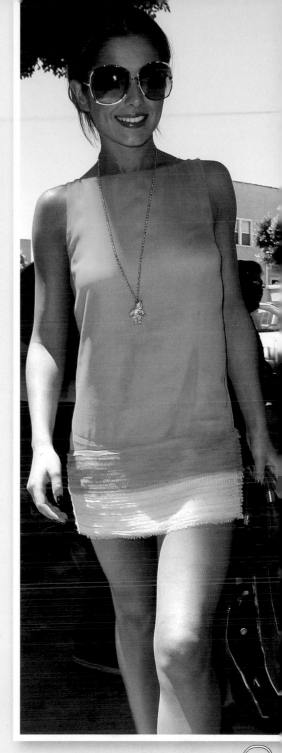

'I've learned how to dress – wearing what suits my shape best.'

Grazia

While some celebrities end up looking older than their years in the quest for style, Cheryl will take classic items such as a fitted jacket or smart shirt, but always add her own twist – a dash of animal print, a brightly coloured oversized bag or a funky waist-length necklace – to keep it age-appropriate.

GIRLS' NIGHT OUT

When Cheryl goes out for a night on the town, the sophisticated lacquer of work and red carpet melts away and she can really cut loose and vamp it up. She favours little dresses and a lot more sex factor than she would usually wear.

For example, for front-row seats at the Julien Macdonald show at London Fashion Week in 2007, she opted for a sheer nude vest over black bra with a pencil skirt and leopard-print skinny belt, while for her twenty-sixth birthday bash in July 2009 she wore a daring slashed-to-the-waist Alexander McQueen dress.

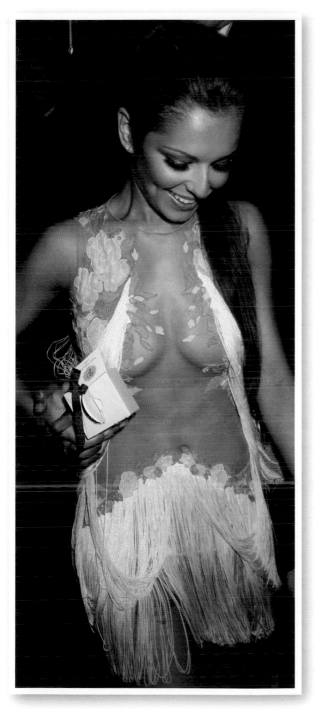

SACK THE STYLIST?

The dress's tasselled skirt drew unflattering comparisons to a 'reworked eighties lampshade' from the *Daily Mail*. However, such negativity doesn't wash with Cheryl. She has regularly spoken about the fact that, even though she has professional stylists on hand as part of her job, she will continue to make her own choices when she's off-duty. She's well aware that, sometimes, people won't like them.

'People have this false idea that we have a machine around us that drives us,' she told *Dreams That Glitter*. 'Sometimes I'll go out and it'll be "Sack the stylist!" Do they really think I got a stylist over just to go out to a club? No. People have this idea everything's controlled and it's not.'

While Cheryl's stylists are on hand for all her work, it's clear that she still makes a lot of her own decisions. And even though there may be the occasional negative review, in truth that epitomizes Cheryl: in the absence of perfection, she may not always get it right – but she's unfailingly herself.

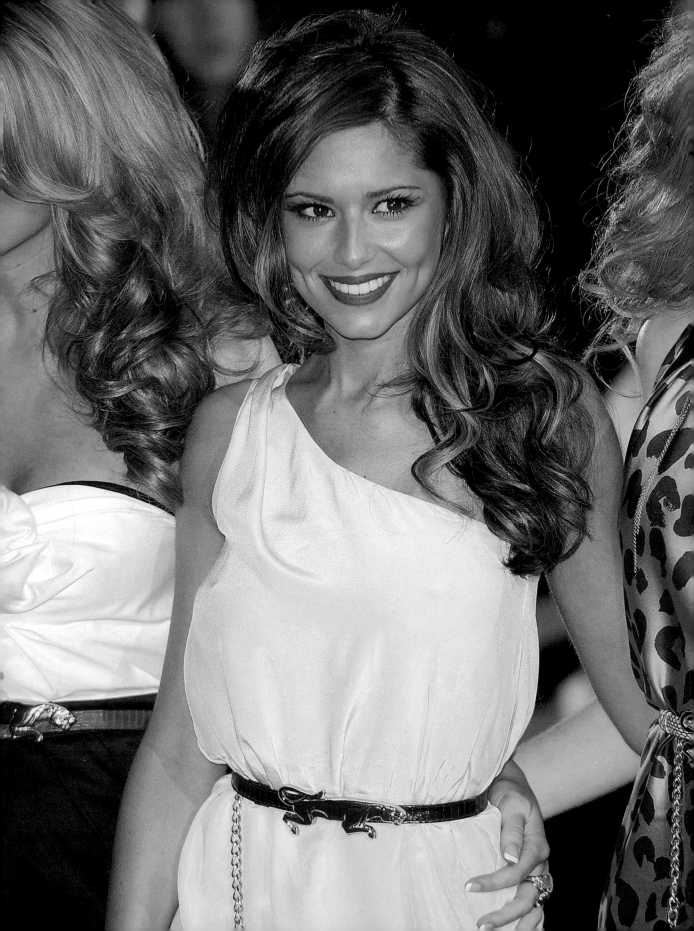

THE STATEMENT DRESS

One of Cheryl's most memorable style phases came at one of the most difficult times in her life.

When it was alleged that husband Ashley had cheated on her with hairdresser Aimee Walton, she became queen of the statement dress, sporting a series of brightly coloured, barely-there frocks which showed her husband exactly what he was missing.

★ A strapless tangerine sheath for a girls' night out in LA.
★ A candy-striped Hervé Léger bandage dress for a trip to top London restaurant Nobu.
★ A canary yellow one-shouldered Alice + Olivia minidress – teamed with a slick of fuchsia lipstick – for the BRIT Awards.

'I like simple. I like matchy. I'm not into clashy.' *Elle*

READ MY CHEST

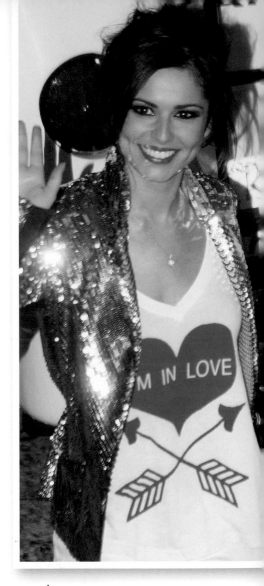

Everyone knows that Cheryl always wears her heart on her sleeve – but recently she has taken to wearing it on her chest, too.

When there were rumours that she and Ashley were having problems in December 2009, she chose fashion to make her statement. She wore a Wildfox T-shirt emblazoned with hearts and the words 'I'm in love', along with a beaming smile and – just in case people didn't get the message – her husband on her arm.

Fast-forward two months and, on the day she announced their separation, she flew to LA wearing a Beatrice Boyle T-shirt featuring a weeping woman, leaving fans in no doubt as to her inner turmoil. A few days later, in the LA sunshine, she chose a significant 'I left my heart in Beverly Hills' T-shirt, also by Wildfox.

While she may not want to get drawn into the mud-slinging of giving statements at certain times, succinct and significant style choices clearly get her message across.

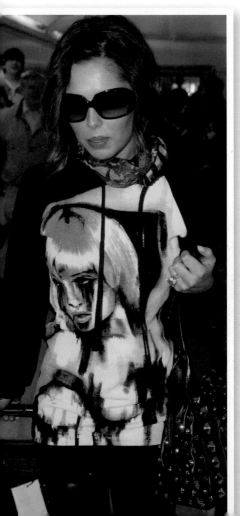

INSIDE CHERYL'S WARDROBE

While the stylish star does sometimes opt for designer labels and haute couture, her wardrobe is more accessible than you might think. Cheryl said in *Girls Aloud Style* that, even after reaching the giddy heights of fame, she still loves high-street stores: 'I like what I like, whether it's Topshop, Miss Selfridge, Prada or Fendi.' And she added in *Dreams That Glitter*, 'If I like something I bought four seasons ago, I'll wear it.'

It took Cheryl a long time to get used to having the money to buy herself nice things. She would frequently feel bad about how much her clothes cost, saying in *Dreams That Glitter*, 'I would buy new clothes and they would stay in the wardrobe. I kept them for "good" like in the old days. I just felt guilty and I struggled to justify spending a large amount of money on things.'

Slowly, Cheryl has adjusted to having the kind of wealth she'd never dared to dream of, and has begun to make the most of what her hard work has given her. 'I've started thinking, you know what, I work hard, I work long hours, I can afford to buy it, and if I want a pair of £300 shoes, I'll get them.'

'I always look on the Topshop website or My-Wardrobe, and net-a-porter.com is right up there.'
Celebs on Sunday

ACCESSORIES

'I'd snap me neck for shoes and handbags.' *Stylist*

HANDBAGS Cheryl always accessorizes her outfits with the hottest outsized bags of the moment, such as the Dolce and Gabbana Lily, Louis Vuitton Monogram and Jimmy Choo Mandah (pictured). She is a huge fan of the huge bag and is usually never without one slung over the crook of her arm.

She told *Glamour* online, 'People often say, "What on earth do you have a handbag *that* size for?" but you'd be surprised what you can fit in it. I get a whole make-up bag in there, serum, some face wipes and, if I'm travelling, I've been known to stuff a pair of shoes in too – I'm not joking!'

She loves bright colours and animal prints, and favours Jimmy Choo for most of her handbag needs, stepping out with a vast array of his range. She opted for an Alexander McQueen when she headed off to Kilimanjaro, and sent a message with a fearsomely studded Christian Louboutin bag after her separation from Ashley.

HATS She frequently plays around with hats and has been spotted in little trilbies and fedoras. On holiday, she'll always plump for a bejewelled straw Stetson.

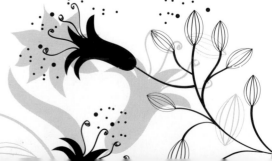

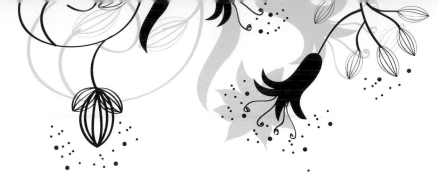

'My all-time favourite item of clothing is high heels. I think high heels can change how you feel as a woman.' *OK!*

SHOES High heels are her favourite part of her wardrobe and – like Sarah Jessica Parker before her – Cheryl loves her Jimmy Choos.

She also favours Rupert Sanderson, but her ultimate favourites are Louboutins: she has often flashed the trademark red sole for both all-out night-time glamour and daytime statement dressing.

SUNGLASSES No celebrity wardrobe would be complete without an array of sunglasses, and Cheryl's is no exception.

She has worn Ray-Bans and DVB from Victoria Beckham's line, but her favourites are by Tom Ford: she has worn countless pairs from his range, including the oversized Bianca, the more delicate Charles, and the funkier, more retro-style Miranda.

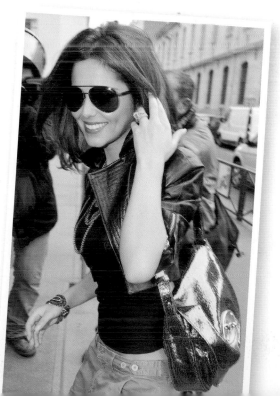

JEWELLERY

For Cheryl, bigger is always better when it comes to jewellery – rings are knuckledusters of diamonds, bracelets are big and chunky, earrings graze her shoulders and necklaces are strung down to her waist.

She said in *Dreams That Glitter*, 'I like big rings, but I'll buy costume jewellery because we get slated if we wear things more than once or twice, so if it's between a pair of 18-carat gold hoop earrings that cost £500, or a pair from Topshop for £3.50, I'll buy the ones from Topshop.'

RINGS
She has a weakness for rings and her more expensive ones boast whopping diamonds – her favourite diamonds are champagne or yellow – but even the less dressy finger bling is still big and flashy.

She's worn huge cocktail rings, and after splitting with Ashley wore first a Bex Rox chunky gold love knot from the Venus range on her wedding finger, followed by an Alexander McQueen skull with red jewels.

BRACELETS
She likes chunky wrist cuffs in black or gold, notably by Mawi or Stephen Webster, and has also worn a pair of chunky silver Bibi charm bracelets that come with hearts, peace signs and car keys already attached.

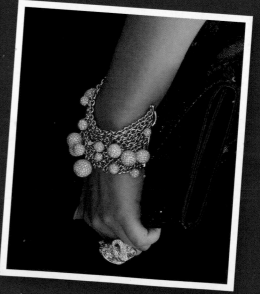

Cheryl loves hearts, and as well as wearing them on T-shirts and charm bracelets, she also likes them in rings and pendants.

NECKLACES

Cheryl has talked about the fact she thinks she can look 'too booby', which is probably why she doesn't wear shorter, dressier necklaces that draw attention to her cleavage.

Instead, she favours long chains with pendants over the top of T-shirts for a more casual look.

EARRINGS

Day or night she likes big statement earrings, and often wears a disco-ball shape that she wore in hot pink for *The X Factor*, silver for *Friday Night with Jonathan Ross*, and coral for a trip to 10 Downing Street.

She also likes long strands with beads by Bex Rox, big jewelled hoops and, for the evening, diamonds down to her shoulders.

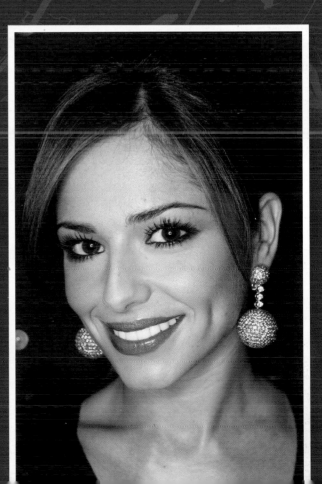

DRESSING FOR HER SHAPE

'I do have a weakness for jackets.' *Dreams That Glitter*

Although a life on the stage requires a lot of skimpy outfits – whether that calls for a skintight catsuit, a slashed-to-the-waist all-in-one, or a micro-mini – it's all part of the job. However, when it's back to reality, Cheryl isn't quite so keen to flash the flesh.

This is something that has come with time. In the early days of her celebrity, she often favoured button-popping shirts and low-cut dresses, but she's since spoken about feeling like her boobs are too big for her frame and so she doesn't usually show off plunging cleavage, preferring higher or square necklines.

She's also spoken many times about her dislike of her legs and although she does sometimes wear miniskirts, she feels safer and more comfortable in jeans and leggings with long T-shirts – always pairing them with her trusty heels to make her look taller.

She has also used cropped jackets over longer tops underneath to give the illusion that her body is longer than it is.

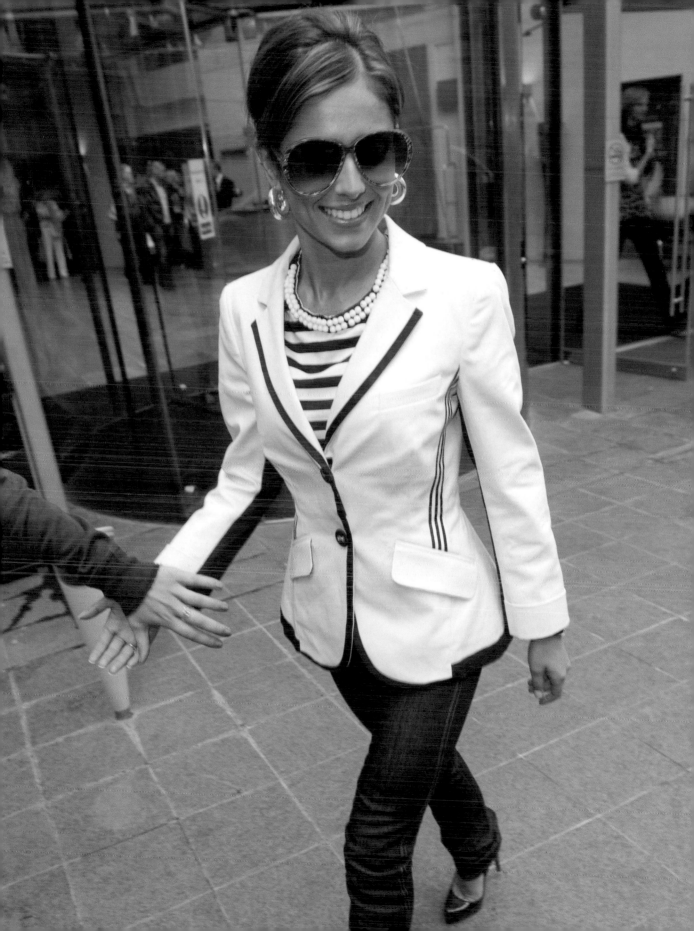

POP PRINCESS

As a pop star, Cheryl has unprecedented access to the hottest new looks and latest fashions. Yet she has to tread a style tightrope, marrying the opinions of stylists with her own ambitions for a fresh new look for each video, tour and album.

In the early days of Girls Aloud, the teenaged Cheryl favoured cornrows, pink Crocs and boob tubes. She said in *Dreams That Glitter*, 'I used to be a bit tomboy-ish and loved trainers, Timberland boots and baggy trousers, so when I got in the band that's what I wanted.'

But as the band evolved into a polished and professional group of young women – in colour-coordinated pencil skirts, with blouses cinched in with big belts for the 'Biology' video – their style savvy matured too. By the time 'The Promise' was released, the girls' gold sequinned fishtail gowns were the envy of women all over the country.

Nearly a decade down the line, Cheryl now has the budget and the clout to do things exactly as she wishes.

'I think your style changes as you get older.' *Dreams That Glitter*

BEHIND THE SCENES

It's in the nature of Cheryl's job that she's expected to look dazzling on all occasions – to be innovative in her fashion choices and to break new ground. A whole team of people have a hand in enabling her to achieve this challenging brief, from the backstage dressers on her tours to the designers who create her show outfits. Cheryl – and Girls Aloud – were assigned two new stylists in 2005, with whom they have worked ever since:

★ **Victoria Adcock**, who has also worked with Victoria Beckham and Christina Aguilera, and who was taken on to move the girls' look away from the high street to something more 'high end'.

★ **Frank Strachan**, who has worked with Kylie Minogue and is about all-out glamour.

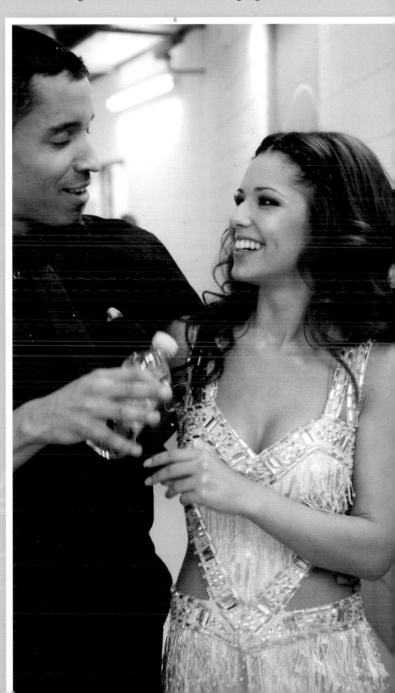

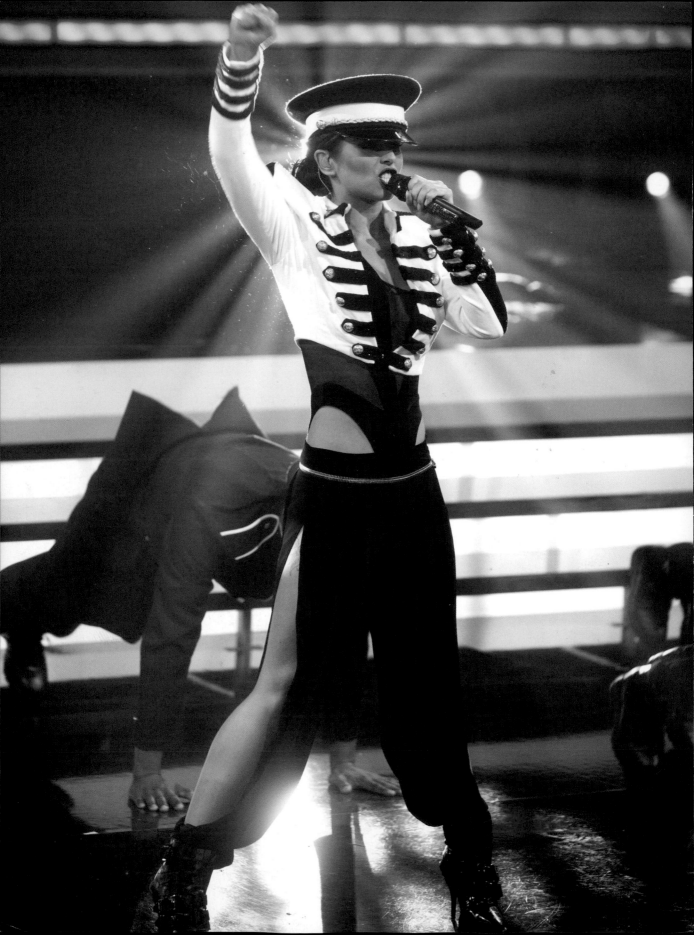

SOLO CHIC

When Cheryl released her debut solo album *3 Words*, and single 'Fight for this Love', in October 2009, she was a seasoned professional in presenting herself in exactly the way she wanted. Opting for a distinctly military ensemble of the soon-to-be-iconic black cap, Balmain red coat and LNA leggings for the video shoot, her look was later reworked by designer Julien Macdonald for her performances on *The X Factor* and Children in Need, among others.

The designer told *Vogue*, 'She called me up and had a few ideas, we went through them and she selected it (the outfit) and absolutely loved it. It was taken from things she loves – she does a lot of dance, so upbeat tracksuit pants with a slash. So when she's dancing, her legs flash through, which is a bit cheeky.

'Underneath is one of my new swimwear pieces. She liked the idea of athletic and swimwear together. And then the military jacket with exaggerated shoulders to give a fashion shoulder. She wanted a hard military look, but wanted it to be current and have a dance energy.'

After Cheryl and Ashley divorced and the song's lyrics took on a new meaning, Cheryl stuck with the military theme, opting for slashed camouflage-patterned harem pants for her performances on tour.

INTRODUCING ...

The 2009 season was when Cheryl started favouring a new designer who swiftly became one of her favourites – Stéphane Rolland.

After wearing three of his designs during the series – a pleat-detail LBD; a gold dress with oversized black bow; and a bespoke gown featuring puffed shoulders, a short hemline and a sweeping train – she also opted for a Rolland gown for the National Television Awards 2010, choosing a stunning silver floor-length dress with matching cuffs.

Cheryl modified the gown from its catwalk incarnation, having the dress fully lined in order to make it a more demure outfit. Previously, it had been a sheer dress from top to toe. She also lost the sleeves from the catwalk version, instead opting for a sleeveless design – although she paired the gown with the dove grey wrist cuffs, which coordinated perfectly and brought a typically Cheryl fashion edge to the whole ensemble.

'I am proud to dress a young beauty like Cheryl.'

Stéphane Rolland, *Now*

Cheryl has said that she would like to sell her *X Factor* outfits and give the proceeds to charity.

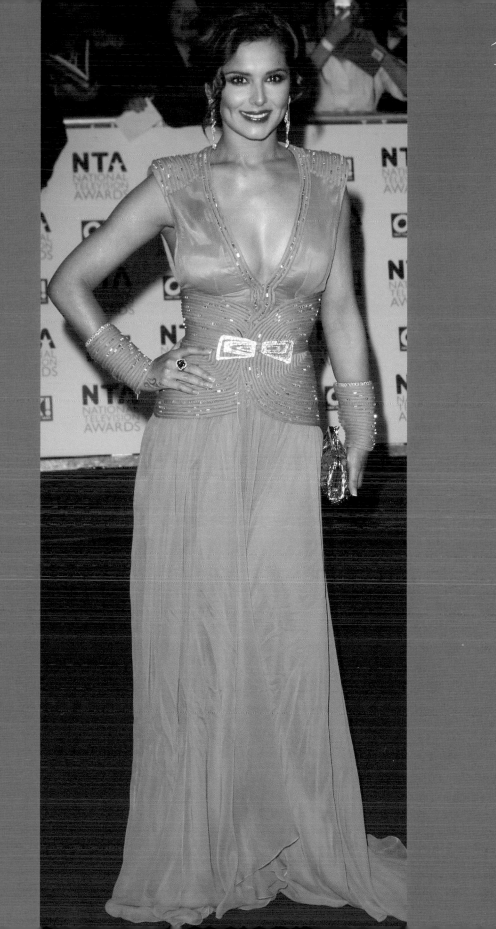

CHERYL'S FAVOURITE DESIGNERS

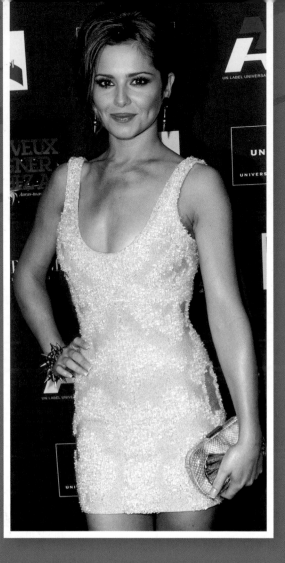

HERVÉ LÉGER

The king of minidresses as far as Cheryl is concerned. He was the man behind her tangerine sheath in LA, as well as her strapless dress for the Starnight awards in Germany, and her silver outfit for the AZ party at the VIP Room in Paris (pictured).

She's also worn him for several nights out at favourite restaurant Nobu.

ALEXANDER MCQUEEN

Cheryl has frequently worn Alexander McQueen: stand-out looks include the sheer black-and-nude top she wore for *X Factor* auditions, her twenty-sixth-birthday frock, and her outfit for her visit to Downing Street.

When he died, she said, 'Fashion has lost one of its most talented and inspirational figures.'

VERSACE

Lampshade dresses on *The X Factor*; Simon Cowell's fiftieth birthday party.

JULIEN MACDONALD

He created the 'Fight for this Love' performance
outfits for *The X Factor* and Children in Need,
and has dressed Cheryl for various *X Factor*
shows, including the first finale. She also wore
him for Gary Barlow's anniversary party, and for
London Fashion Week (pictured).

Julien told *Vogue*: 'I've been working
with Cheryl for a long time, she's attended my
shows and we've formed a friendship.'

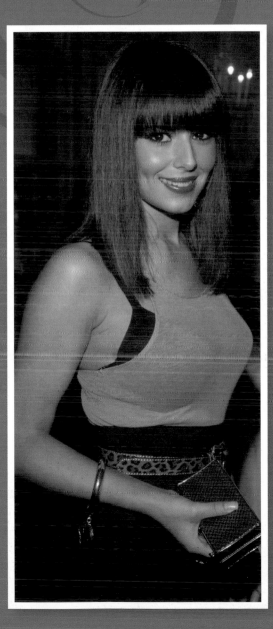

Lots of *X Factor*, and the National Television
Awards 2010.

MATTHEW WILLIAMSON

The National Television Awards 2008; many
X Factor shows. Cheryl was also photographed
with him in his store.

FASHION FORWARD

'I would love my own clothing range.' MySpace

Cheryl is not one to rest on her fashion laurels and has revealed in a live MySpace chat, 'I would love my own clothing range, but if I did ever do it, I would like to put the time and effort in properly and do the whole thing myself.

'It would probably be a high-street collection. I would take inspiration from designer stuff, but turn it into high street.'

Celebrity stylist Hannah Sandling told documentary *Changing Faces – Cheryl Cole*, 'I think we need to watch closely because we've seen people like Victoria Beckham bring out various labels, we've seen people like Kate Moss. I hope she's going to be the next girl because I tell you this – what she designs, everybody's going to be buying into it.'

As Cheryl's boss and friend Simon Cowell is big buddies with businessman Philip Green, who owns the Arcadia Group (which includes Topshop, Miss Selfridge and Dorothy Perkins), it's not impossible to imagine she may hook up professionally with the retail giant one day.

It seems it's just a case of finding the time to fit it in – along with working on a flourishing solo career, continuing her commitments with Girls Aloud, doing more television and charity work ... and general world domination!

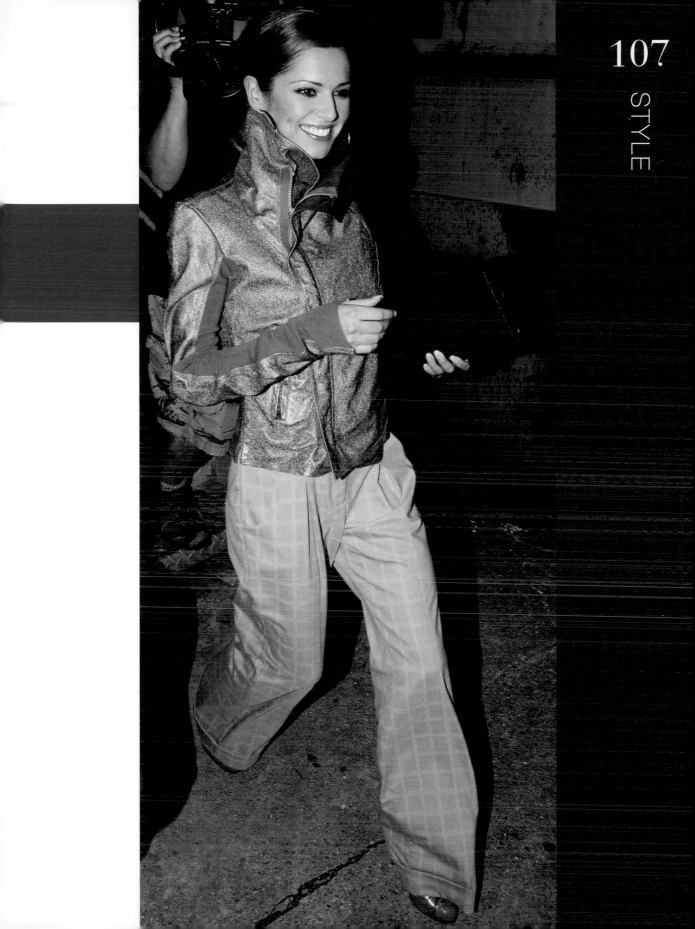

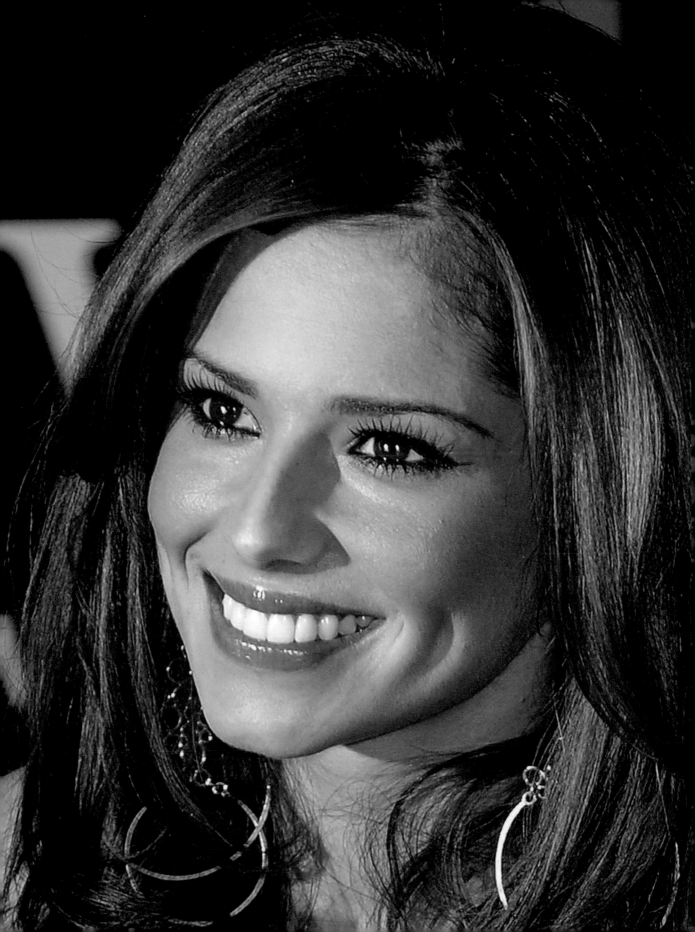

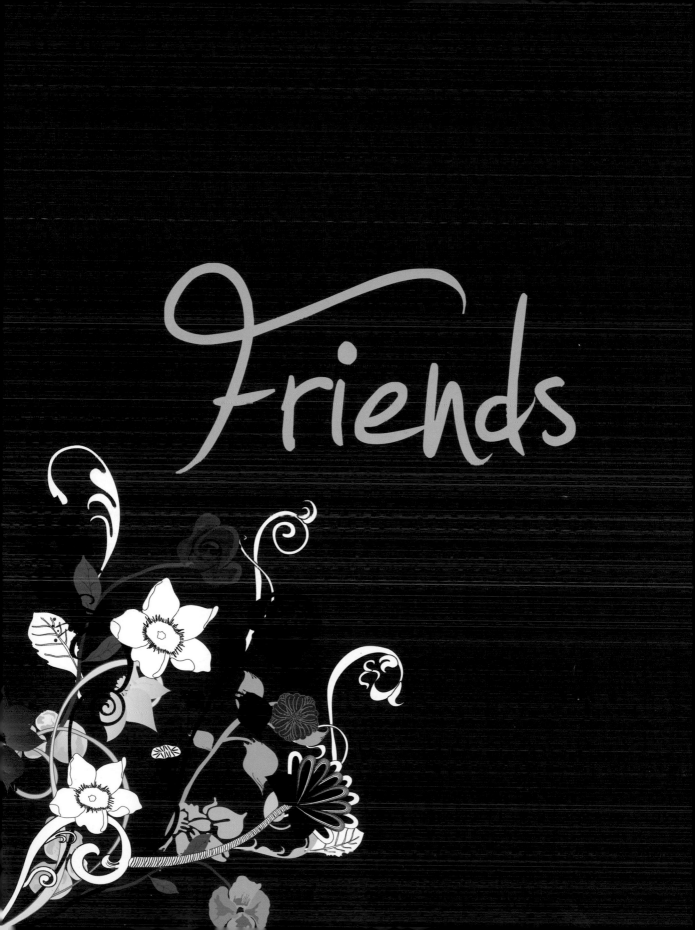

'Trust is so important to me.'

OK!

Despite having the kind of lads'-mag-poll-topping looks that could easily scare off other girls, Cheryl has a tight clique of female friends and is a true girl's girl. She really values the importance of female relationships, telling *Elle* magazine, 'Imagine that you had no girlfriends. You're in the shit. Men don't understand hormones. We need each other.'

While some attractive women in the public eye cultivate an image as red-hot and sexy as possible – scaring off both female fans and potential friends alike – Cheryl plays down her physical attributes and is quick with a self-deprecating remark or a no-nonsense opinion that endears her to both sexes.

Whether it's chart rivals, older colleagues or the new generation of female stars – there's plenty of Cheryl-love to go around when it comes to her friendships.

BEING CHERYL

110

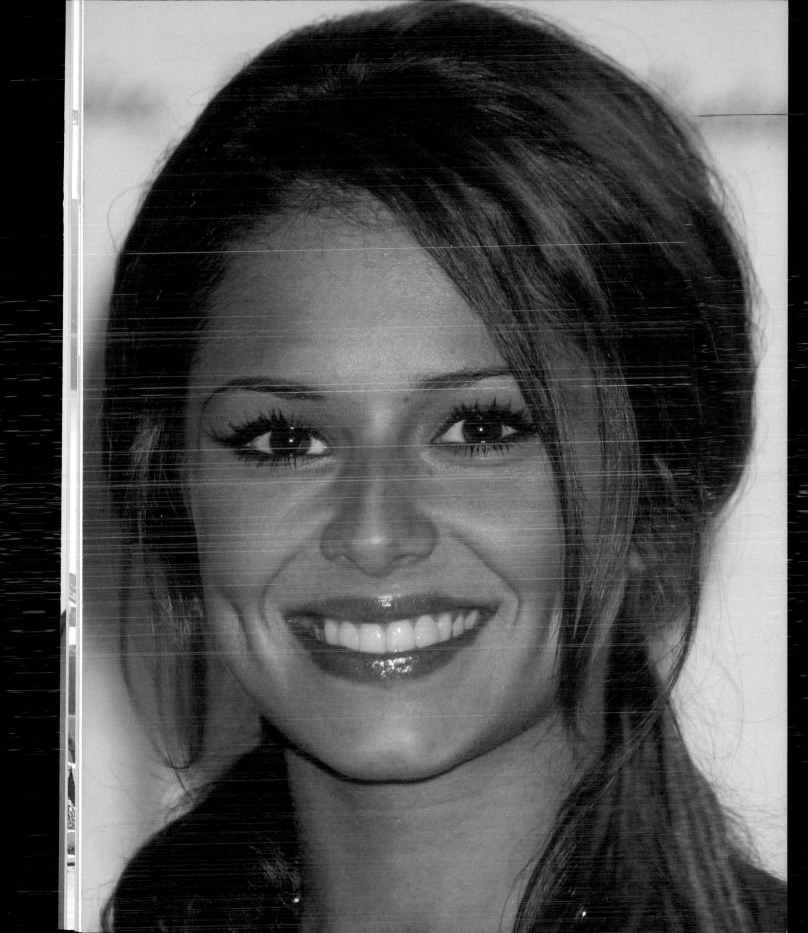

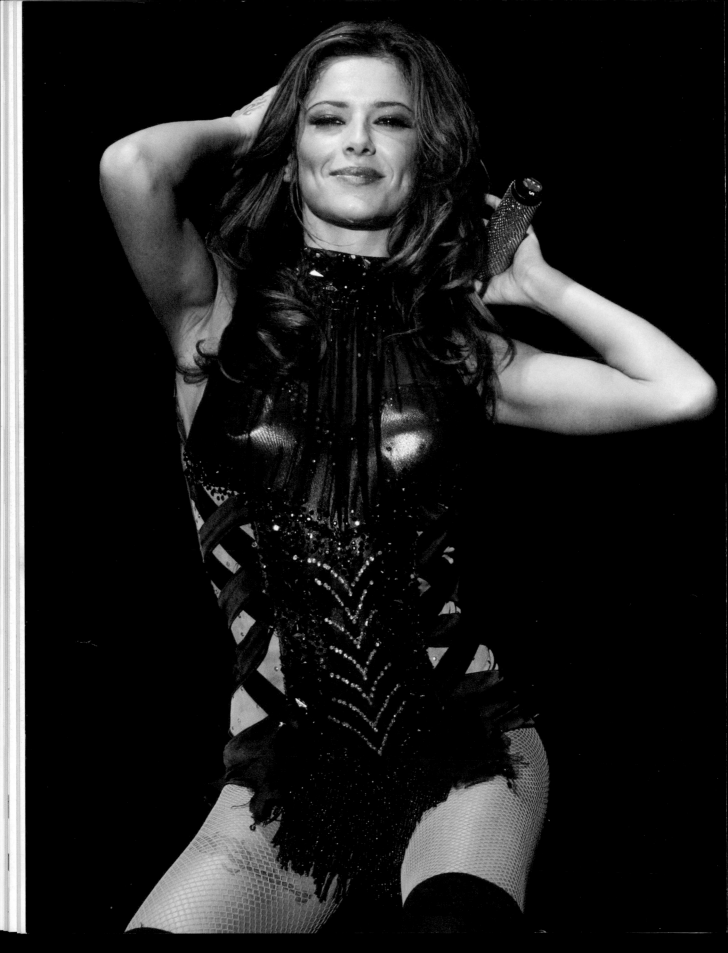

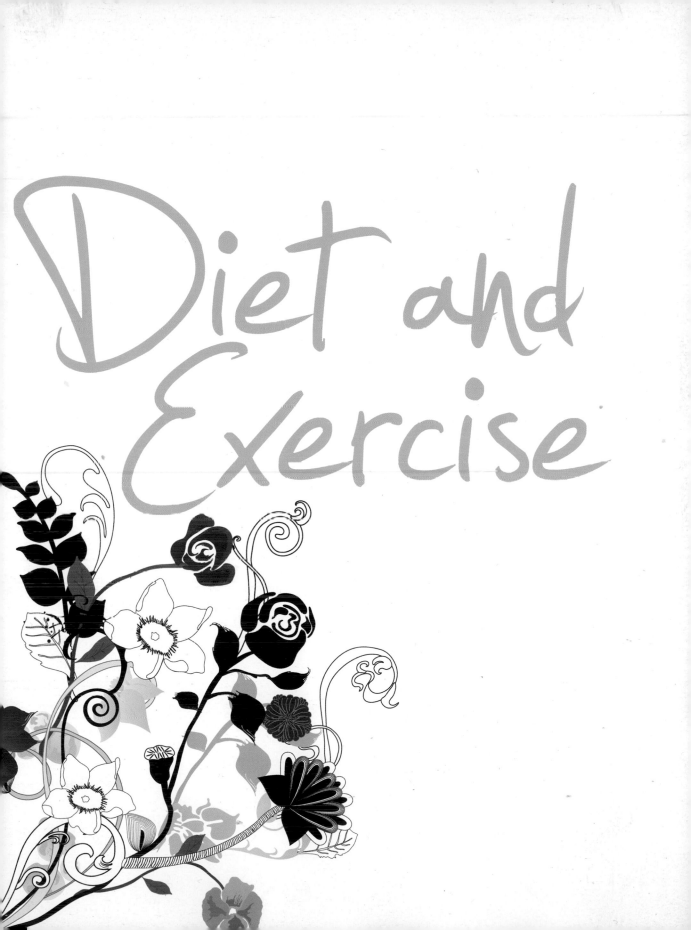

Diet and Exercise

When your job is 'pop star', the lifestyle ranges from relentless physical activity whilst touring – performing onstage every night and rehearsing during the day – to lots of sitting around whilst recording, confined to the same place for long hours; and then whatever the hell you want when you have some rare time off.

However, when your schedule is combined with a TV career that means criss-crossing the country for auditions in different cities, and then spending whole evenings in a vast studio with whatever catering is provided, it means that doing a weekly grocery shop or keeping up the gym membership becomes something of a problem.

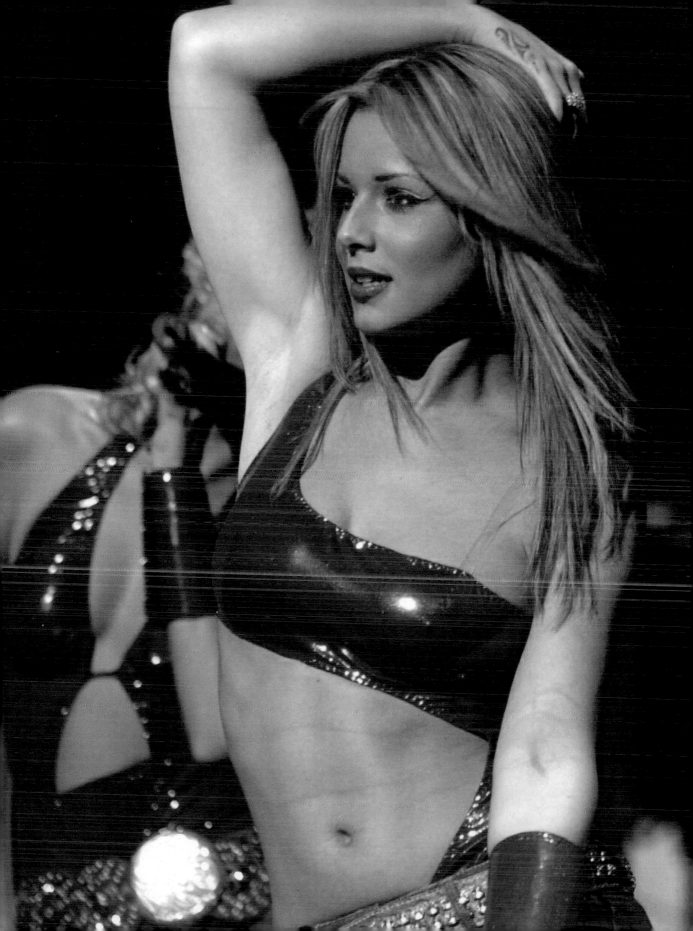

PINT-SIZE PRINCESS

Cheryl's weight has fluctuated slightly over the years and a lot has been said about her size, but for anyone in any doubt that she is a healthy and natural weight for her five-foot-three-inch frame, they need look no further than her mother Joan. Even shorter than her diminutive daughter and with similar measurements, it's obvious that a petite physique is simply in the genes – although that doesn't make for interesting tabloid reading ...

Whilst equally tiny stars such as Kylie Minogue and Sienna Miller have been celebrated as pocket sex bombs and not had to face scrutiny about their dinky proportions, Cheryl is often under the media microscope about her weight.

So how *does* she stay so trim? She says it's a combination of good metabolism and healthy diet, but even though she has now trained herself to develop the eating habits of a sophisticated young woman, she still sometimes reverts back to the basic tastes of the proverbial kid in a sweet shop ...

CHERYL'S FAVOURITE FOODS

★ Japanese food – sushi, miso soup, tempura
★ Italian food – spaghetti bolognese, lasagne
★ Fish and seafood
★ Steak and chips

FISH FINGERS TO ROCK SHRIMP

Cheryl grew up with little money and no knowledge of healthy eating, saying that she and her family lived mainly on fish fingers, beans and bread, but over the years she has broadened her horizons with different kinds of food. She's said she would never have tried an olive before and now loves them, but she still doesn't like goat's cheese.

'I hated fish and seafood,' she revealed in *Dreams That Glitter*. 'Now I'll eat smoked haddock, cod and shrimp. I eat vegetable sushi and I've tried rock shrimp, but I soak it in soy sauce. I love tempura, miso soup and edamame beans.'

Her bandmate Kimberley Walsh also revealed that Cheryl likes cherry tomatoes dipped in salt as a snack.

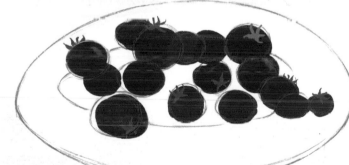

'I've got a real thing about salt. I put it on everything.'

Dreams That Glitter

BALANCED DIET

Cheryl's eating habits have completely changed from her early days in the band, when she shared a flat with Nicola Roberts and lived on junk food.

'We didn't ever cook, just lived on noodles and beans and bacon butties and takeaways: Domino's pizza, wedges and garlic dip every night,' Nicola revealed in *Dreams That Glitter*. 'There were pizza boxes everywhere.'

These days, Cheryl simply sticks to a balanced diet – sometimes she has salad, sometimes she has fish and chips. Her menu, however, often depends on where she is.

Like everyone, she's dictated to by work. Some people grab a piece of toast on their way to the office or eat lunch at their desk; for Cheryl, there's a lot more travel involved, but it's much the same principle. She is often zipping all over the world thanks to her music and TV work, and it's difficult to keep up any kind of healthy eating when you wake up in different cities every day and different time zones are confusing your body clock.

FAVOURITE FOODS

Cheryl likes traditional, simple fare. At her wedding, the menu was prawn cocktail starters and a main of steak and chips, followed by miniature banoffi pies, while backstage at the V Festival in 2008 she requested fried chicken, cornbread, sweet potato mash, green beans and waffles.

She's also a fan of Japanese food, which is healthy and low in fat, and classic Italian dishes, especially spaghetti bolognese and lasagne. Ashley revealed to *Vogue* that she makes good pasta dishes. However, Cheryl is the first to admit that cooking isn't her greatest skill. Consequently, the singer still opts for the odd takeaway.

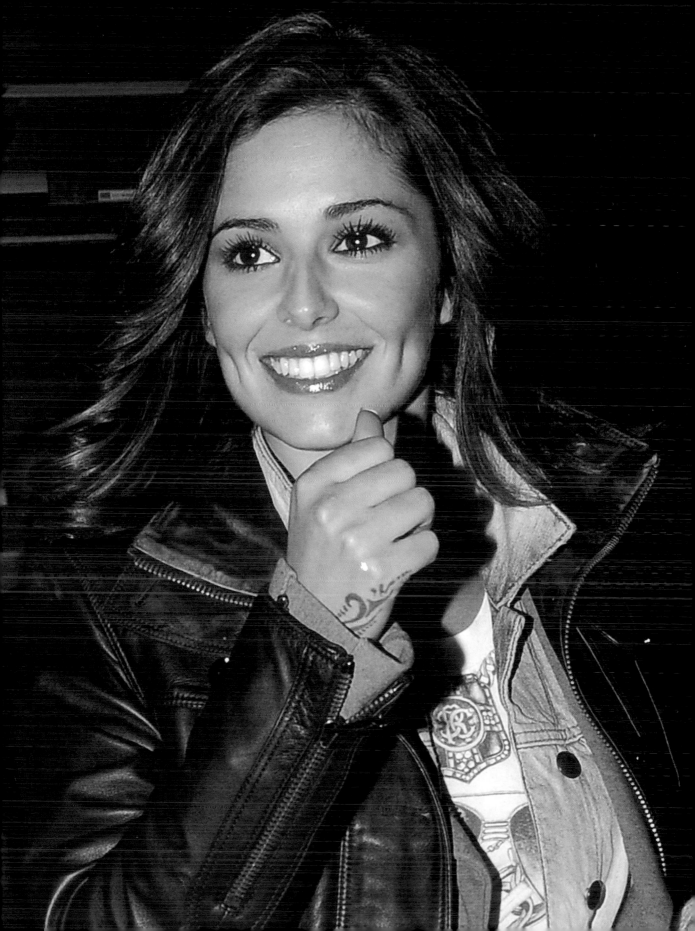

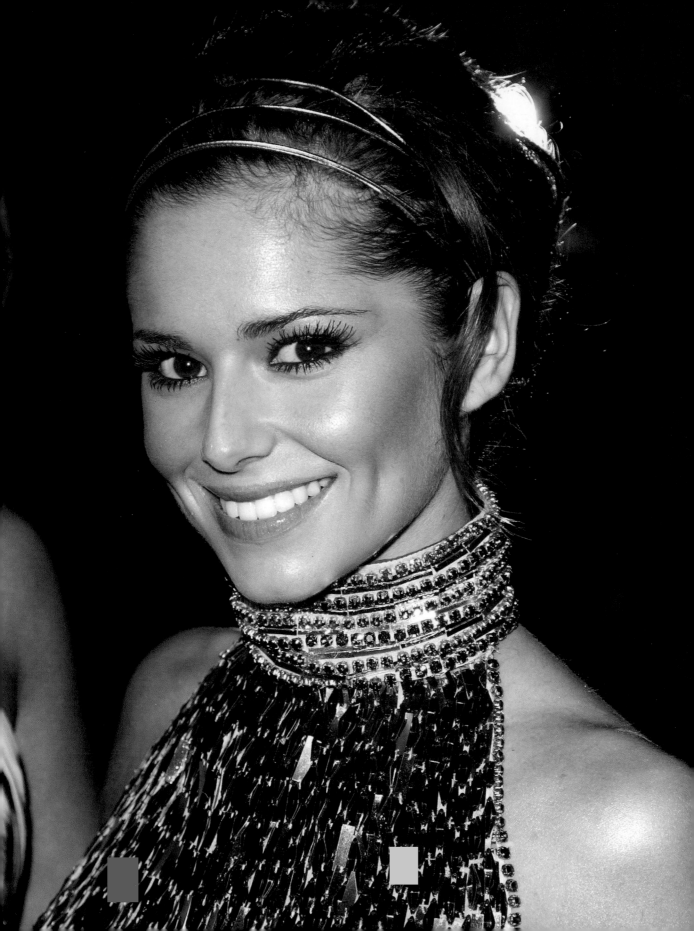

'DIET' IS A FOUR-LETTER WORD

'It annoys me when people say, "Eat this, eat that." If you want it, eat it. Just get off your arse and exercise.'

Now online

After all those pizzas with Nicola, Cheryl's weight went up to nine and a half stone. She tried to lose weight on a fad diet, explaining to *Vogue*, 'Jennifer Aniston was doing something called the Atkins diet and I thought I'd give it a try.'

Girls Aloud were staying in a hotel at the time so she ordered chicken in cream sauce with carrots every night for weeks, adding, 'I just felt horrible.'

Since then, she has avoided gimmicky methods of losing weight, but she did recently try the blood-type diet for an energy boost. Her mum recommended the regime to her and Cheryl told *Hello!*, 'It has made such a difference – not to my shape, but to how I feel and my energy levels. I used to be "energy schmenergy" and I didn't believe it. But now I've done it, I believe it 100 per cent.'

As a general rule, Cheryl says that if she starts the day eating protein, then she tries not to eat carbohydrates.

In short, Cheryl loves her food, doesn't diet, and doesn't have a nutritionist, but simply tries to eat as healthily as possible.

JUST DANCE

Cheryl's background is in dance and it's something she has been passionate about since she was a little girl – even studying at ballet school down in London at the age of eleven.

Effectively, she has been training for most of her life and it means that she has muscle memory, which gives her good foundations for a great physique.

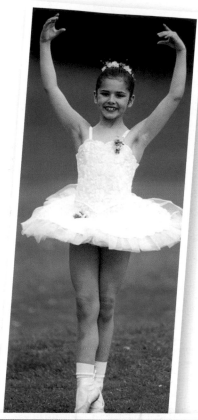

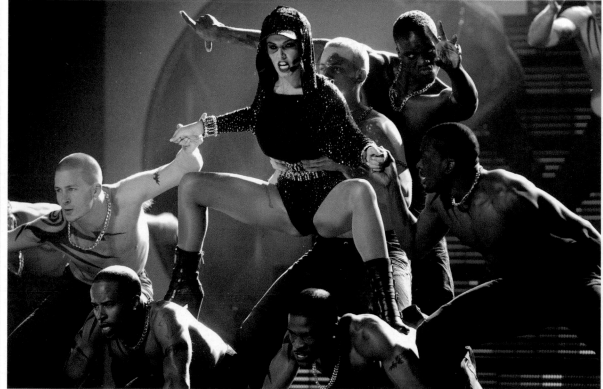

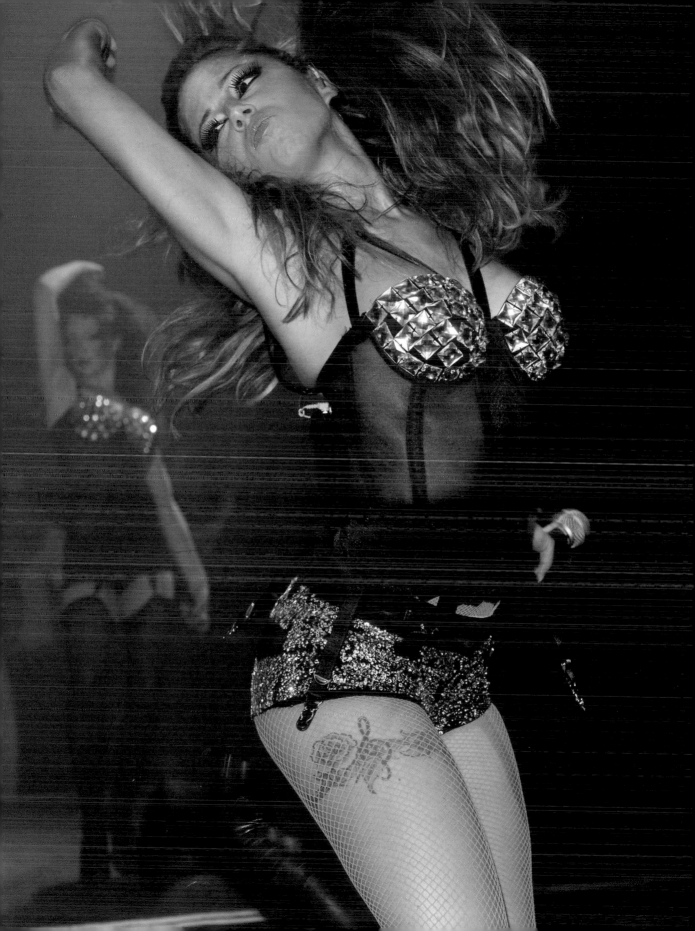

> ## 'I hate looking thin. I don't want to be up and down like a lollipop lady.' *Grazia*

FINDING WHAT WORKS FOR YOU

Like many women, Cheryl has experimented with different ways of staying in shape over the years.

In the early days, when Girls Aloud put on a bit of puppy fat after living alone for the first time and surviving on junk food, they employed a personal trainer and Cheryl told *Now* online, 'I'd go on the treadmill for thirty minutes and then do an hour of resistance work with weights.'

After that, however, she used a hypoxi-machine that she kept at home and later replaced with a wind-tunnel exercise bike.

> These machines work by combining exercise with vacuum pressure to increase the circulation and get rid of fatty tissue.

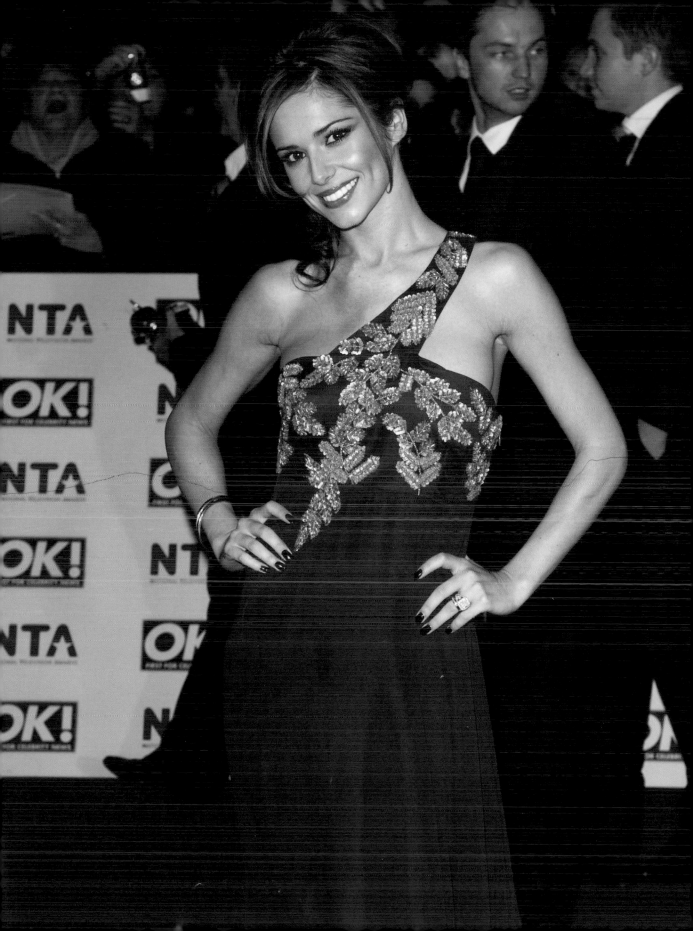

MAINTAINING PHYSIQUE

Luckily for Cheryl, she mainly keeps in shape because of her workload, telling *OK!* magazine, 'If I'm going on tour then I have gruelling schedules and gruelling dance routines. Sometimes I can be dancing for eight hours a day.'

Yet touring takes up only a few months of the year and Cheryl's fitness levels need to be maintained at all times, as it's impossible to sustain a rigorous workload if you're not in tip-top health – plus you never know when you'll need to slip into a little sparkly something and flash the toned flesh for an awards show, charity appearance or photo shoot …

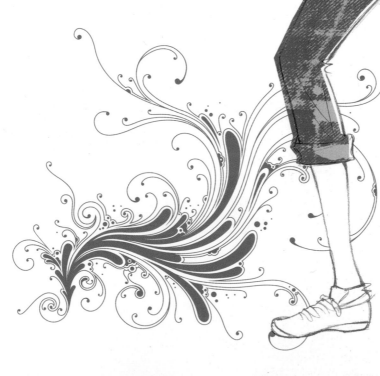

As with most things, there's no secret miracle: she simply maintains her physique with a healthy, active workload. Even when she's not touring, she will still be performing tracks as part of promotion, which often involves blood-pumping dance routines – from the energy of 'Fight for this Love' to the precise ballroom-style choreography of 'Parachute'.

In addition, the activities she chooses when she's not focusing on rehearsing and performing are also pretty arduous – learning how to street-dance for the TV show *The Passions of ... Girls Aloud*, or climbing Mount Kilimanjaro for Comic Relief.

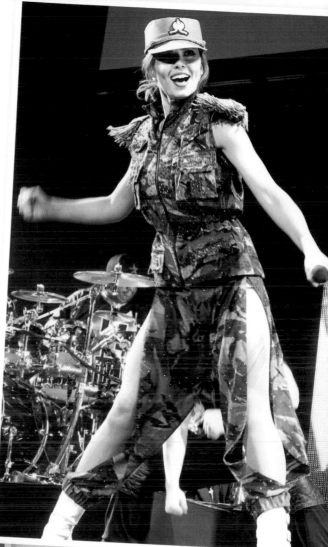

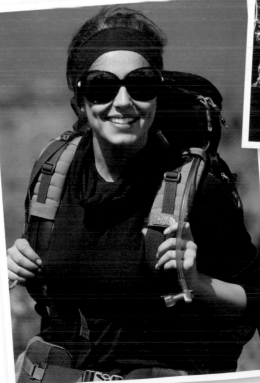

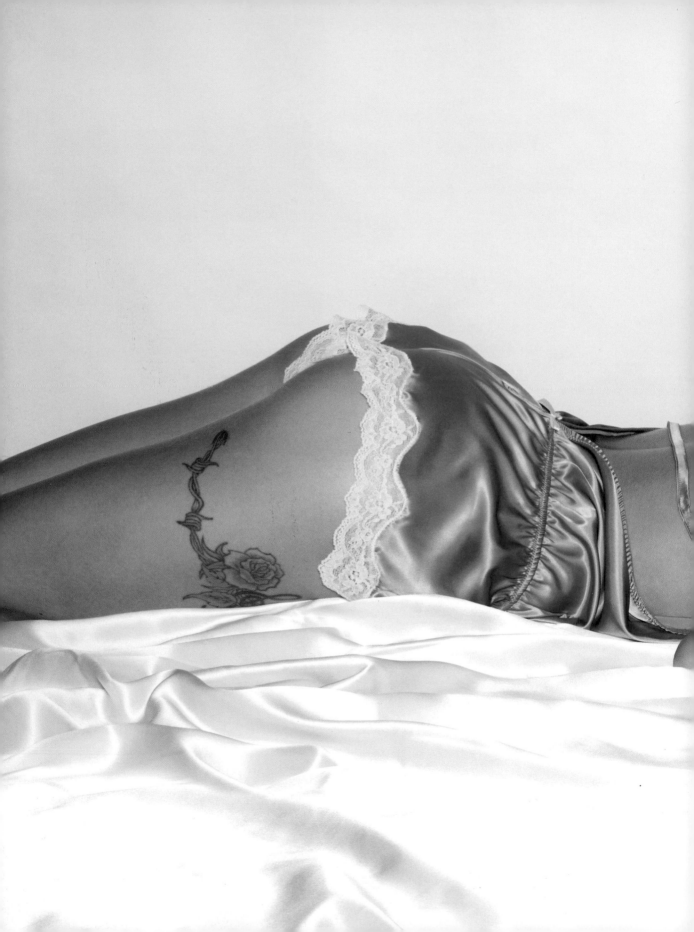

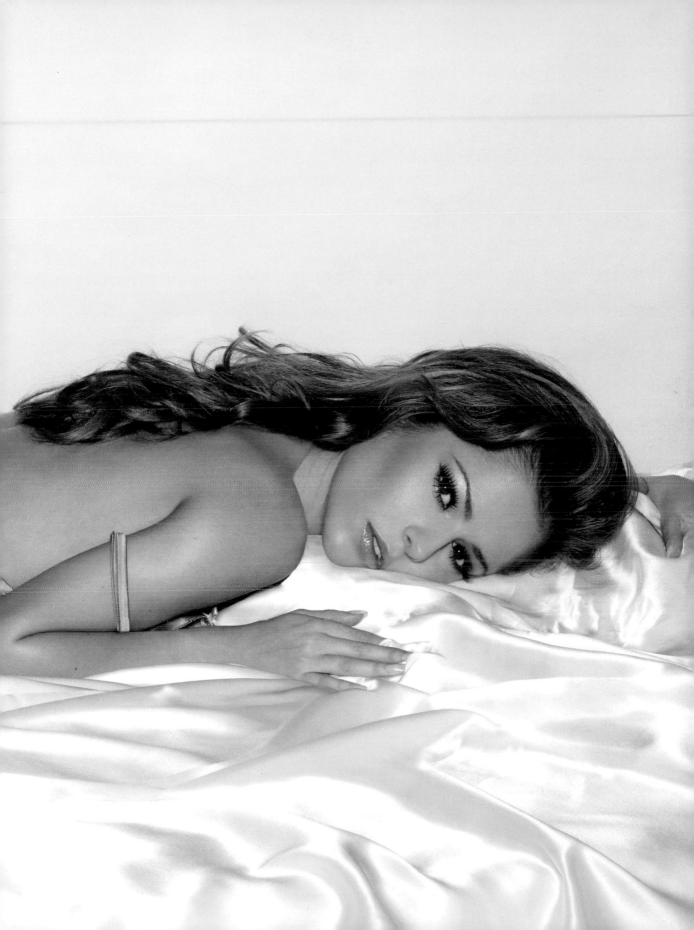

BODY IMAGE

Most women have a love/hate relationship with the way they look, and Cheryl is no different. She has in the past complained about her legs and said she thinks her boobs are too big and her bum is too small, but as she gets older, she has become more accepting, and won't complain about what she perceives to be her physical shortcomings any more. This has a lot to do with wanting to present a positive message to young girls.

In the past, she told *Heat* magazine, 'I don't like my legs. I haven't got much of them for a start.' Adding to the *Mirror*, 'Sometimes I think they are a bit fat, but I know they're not. It's just a complex I've got.'

Cheryl has revealed she used to try all sorts of things in an attempt to change the shape of her legs, such as different kinds of exercise machines and Pilates, but none of them made any difference, so she has come to appreciate what she has and be grateful that she has a pair of working legs.

And that's typical Cheryl – women everywhere can understand what it's like to have personal insecurities, but she works hard to become more at ease with herself and to be an inspiration to the girls who look up to her.

'As a woman, you're never going to be 100-per-cent satisfied. I'm just grateful for the good things.' *Dreams That Glitter*

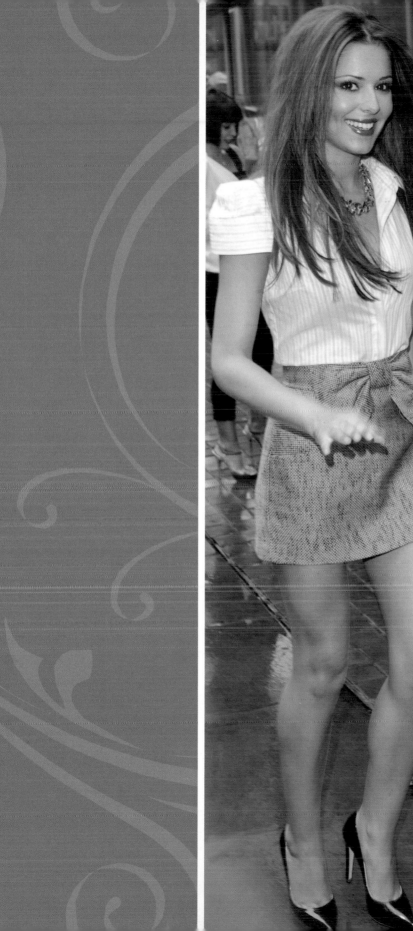

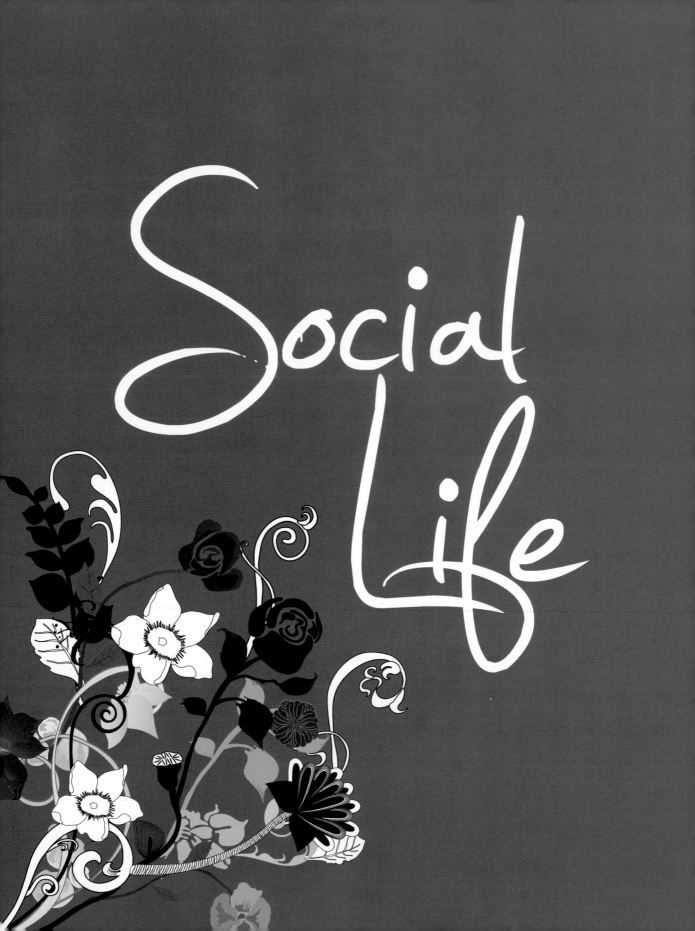

Social Life

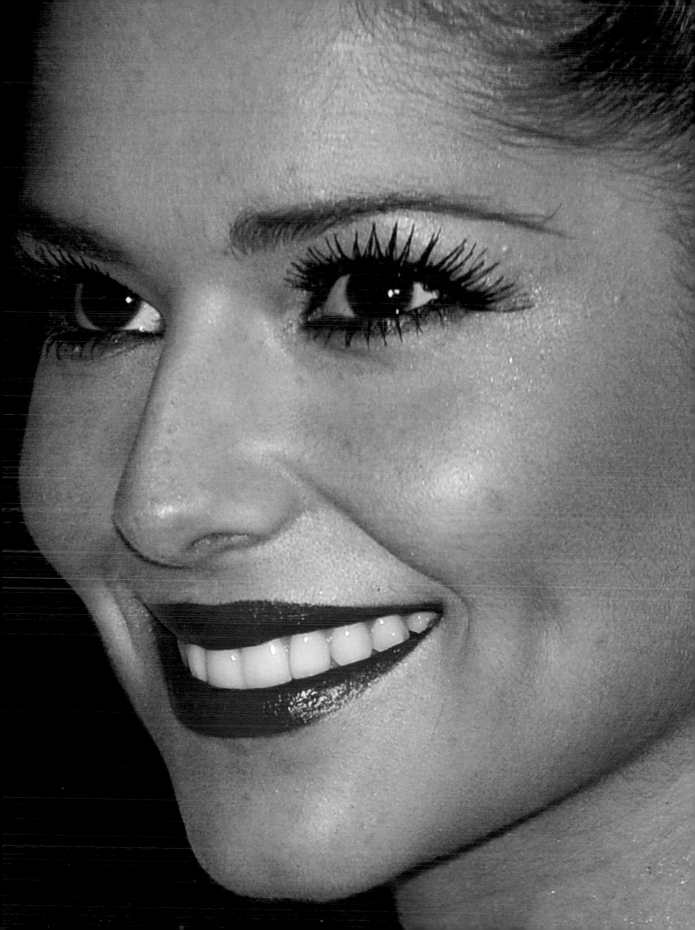

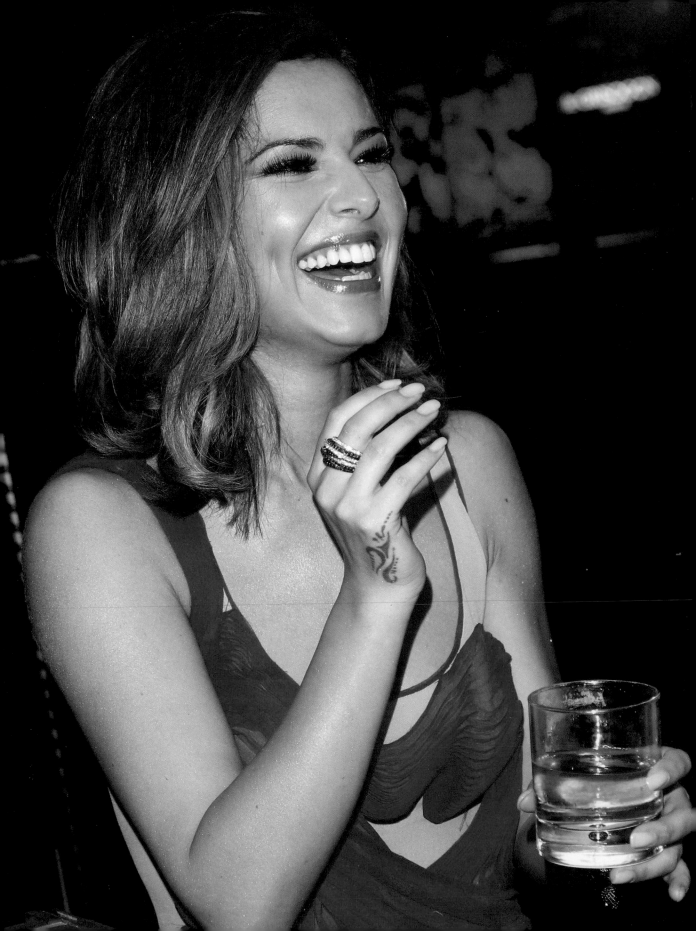

When Cheryl was first on the London party scene with Girls Aloud, she made the most of the fact that she was young, free and single, kicking up her heels in a number of big flashy clubs in London's West End – like Tantra, Chinawhite and Embassy – and she and her bandmates acquired a reputation for partying hard.

However, Cheryl's tastes have since become more discerning. She now favours classic restaurants, hotel bars and private members' clubs in upmarket areas of London for her nights out – opting for drinks or dinner with friends rather than all-night clubbing sessions – or enjoys the thrill of attending concerts by her favourite performers, like Beyoncé, John Legend or Lady Gaga.

In addition, she always makes an effort to attend parties to mark special occasions and was there for Simon Cowell when he turned fifty, for Gary Barlow when he hosted a party to celebrate his ten-year wedding anniversary, and she's always on hand for the birthday parties of close friends and family too.

Cheryl's favourite tipple is champagne; she especially likes pink champagne, opting for Laurent-Perrier rosé at her wedding.

COME DINE WITH ME

Having been brought up with very little money and a limited diet, Cheryl has spoken about how she now has unprecedented opportunities to experiment with different kinds of food, developing a taste for seafood and Japanese cuisine.

She said in *Dreams That Glitter*, 'I remember going to a really posh restaurant in London – Zilli Fish – with the record company to celebrate getting to number one with "Sound of the Underground" and thinking, "There's nothing worse than posh food."'

It's a long time since that night in Zilli Fish, and Cheryl has since made the most of getting to know all the top restaurants in the major cities around the world.

Cheryl celebrated her twenty-fifth birthday in Wing's Chinese restaurant in Manchester. The restaurant is often credited with being one of the finest in the city.

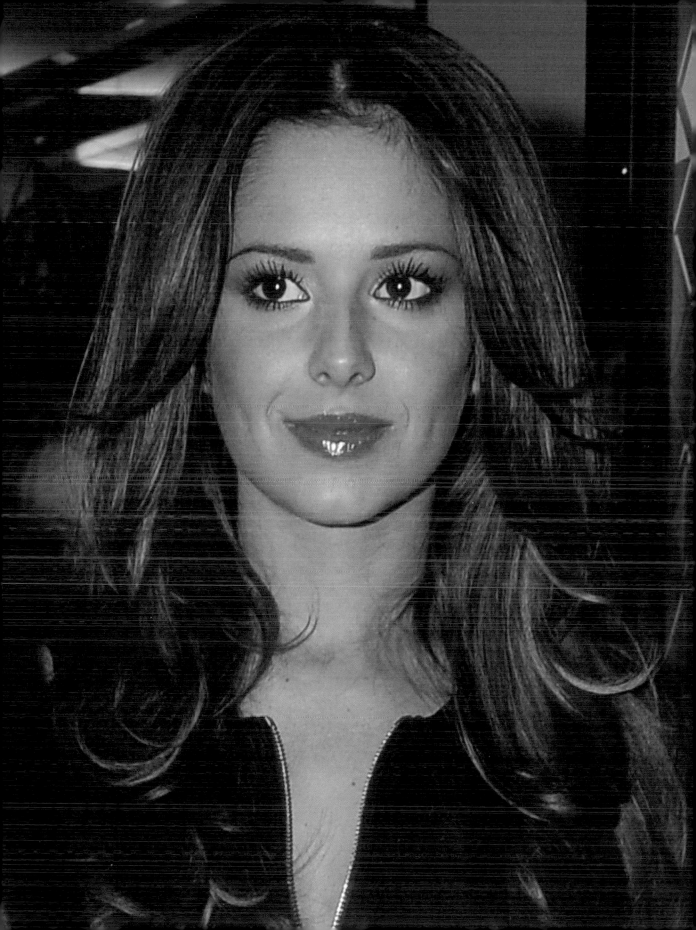

LONDON

Cheryl does most of her socializing in London, as it's the nearest big city to her home in Surrey and she's often there for work or to see friends, so she has a few favourite places she likes to frequent.

She's drawn to distinguished venues that often have a lot of showbiz history attached to them – and it doesn't hurt that they are renowned for their good food, excellent service and discreet treatment of people in the public eye.

NOBU BERKELEY

Her all-time favourite London restaurant is Nobu Berkeley, which is a long-standing celebrity haunt serving Asian food and specializing in rock shrimp tempura and melt-in-the-mouth black cod.

It's light and airy, decorated with silvery tree branches and little white lights, and a very 'celeb' place to go, favoured by Madonna, Gwyneth Paltrow, Kate Moss, Jenson Button, Beyoncé … and the list goes on.

'It's got that romance about it,' Cheryl told *Elle*.

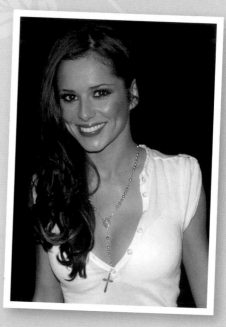

THE IVY

Another classic haunt that she favours is posh but relaxed theatreland favourite The Ivy, which serves up good quality comfort food like the signature salmon fishcakes or sticky toffee pudding.

It is so popular with celebrities that there is a constant gaggle of paparazzi stationed outside throughout the day and night.

THE WOLSELEY

During her first series of *The X Factor*, Cheryl took Alexandra Burke and Diana Vickers to dinner at The Wolseley, which is a grand Italian-style listed building. It serves a European menu, ranging from Black Velvet with oysters, to lamb chops with bubble and squeak, to German sausages.

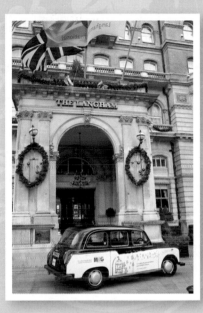

THE LANGHAM HOTEL

Cheryl also likes the traditional feel of the old London hotels. She recently spent an evening with Kimberley and Nicola at the Langham Hotel, a recently refurbished Victorian-era establishment.

Their night out took place the day before she performed on Fearne Cotton's BBC Radio 1 Live Lounge, and Cheryl blamed their evening for the raging hangover she had the next day!

OTHER OLD-SCHOOL FAVOURITES

- ★ Cipriani – an Italian restaurant known for its Bellinis.
- ★ Mr Chow's – an upscale Chinese restaurant that's a favourite of Simon Cowell.
- ★ Zuma – a Knightsbridge hotspot serving contemporary Japanese cuisine.

LA

Now Cheryl has become a transatlantic star, she is finding her feet in Hollywood too – and has been spotted at a few of these premier locations.

CHATEAU MARMONT

Dinner at the Chateau Marmont is always a favourite with celebrities, partly because of their strict 'no cameras allowed' policy (even guests will be asked to put their cameras away if they're spotted), and partly because the very air is infused with Hollywood myth and legend …

The faux French chateau is where James Dean auditioned for *Rebel Without a Cause*, Marilyn Monroe rented a bungalow, Greta Garbo checked in when she wanted 'to be alone' and Jean Harlow honeymooned. It's also where Jim Morrison hurt his back swinging from a window, John Belushi died from a drugs overdose – and Led Zeppelin rode their motorbikes through the lobby.

It still draws the latest hot young stars like Robert Pattinson, Scarlett Johansson, Rihanna and Sienna Miller, who soak up the ambience in the courtyard, sitting in wicker chairs at tables lit with little lamps. Cheryl ate there with friends.

HOUSTON'S

She's been spotted in Houston's in Century City, which is a kitsch seventies-style steakhouse – showing that even though she has become a fan of low-fat, healthy Japanese cuisine, she still likes her hearty fare.

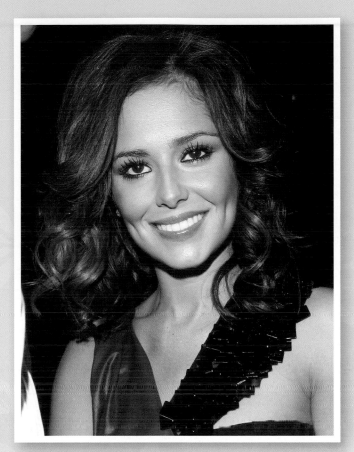

KATSUYA

Cheryl has been for dinner at Japanese restaurant Katsuya on Hollywood Boulevard with Derek Hough and a few pals. They ordered creamy rock shrimp, seared tuna, Japanese salsa, miso-marinated black cod and Kobe tobanyaki.

EUROPE

When Cheryl was in Baden-Baden for the 2006 World Cup, she and Victoria Beckham had an evening meal in Italian restaurant Medici.

During her promotional tour in spring 2010, meanwhile, she went for dinner in top Parisian restaurants Pershing Hall and Hotel Costes.

STARS IN BARS

'I used to love going to parties and clubs, but I think I've grown out of it now.' *The Sun*

Bars are not really Cheryl's scene any more, and she told *The Sun*, 'I got bored of going to the same places, seeing the same people. It doesn't interest me any more. I don't like being drunk and losing control of what I'm saying or doing.'

She told *OK!* magazine that when she does go out, she doesn't feel like it's her vibe now, explaining: 'I'm there looking around and I'm just thinking, "This is not for me." I would rather be at home watching the telly with a takeaway.'

Nevertheless, Cheryl does make an exception sometimes. When she ventures out these days, she tends to opt for hotel bars, as she loves the distinguished feel of these places. For example, she's been to the Mayfair Hotel in London for pre-dinner drinks on a number of occasions. It has recently been refurbished and become a swift favourite celebrity hangout, thanks to the gourmet restaurant and luxurious dark gold and purple décor.

Cheryl also attended Gary Barlow's tenth wedding-anniversary party at the Mandarin Oriental, an old-school favourite on London's Park Lane in Knightsbridge. The Mandarin is another traditional, luxury venue, which has been visited by the Queen, Shirley Bassey, Joan Collins … and now Cheryl too!

IN THE CLUBS

In the past, fun-loving Cheryl chose to celebrate key moments of her life in the capital's top nightspots:

★ In 2005, she held her twenty-second birthday celebrations in London superclub Chinawhite. Back then, it was the stomping ground of glamour models and reality-TV-show contestants, but with its oriental ambience, burning incense, star-cloth ceiling and in-house tarot-reader, it epitomized West End glamour to the young Cheryl.

★ For her hen night, she spent the night in African-themed Umbaba, which has cocktails named after African flowers, colander lampshades in the loos and a safari-themed VIP area.

★ When 'The Promise' got to number one, the girls celebrated in Caribbean-themed Kitts, which has also been a favourite with Prince Harry.

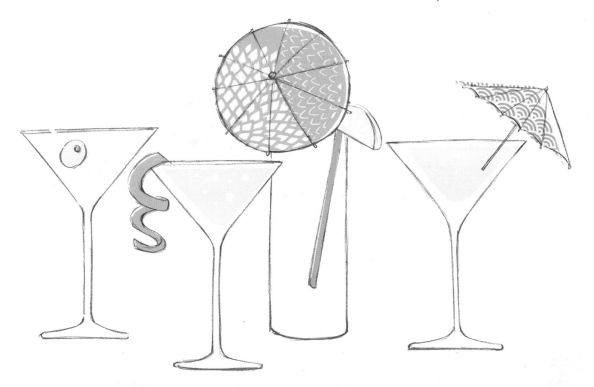

PRIVATE MEMBERS' CLUBS

In recent years, Cheryl has preferred less themed and colourful venues and opted for more subtle places with either a traditional feel or a minimalist vibe. Most of the parties she goes to now are held in private members' clubs, with Nicola's twenty-third birthday party being held at the Wellington Club (pictured).

Often a shroud of secrecy surrounds private members' clubs, as only those with enough money to afford the annual fees – or who know someone who can – will ever get to step inside. The Wellington is old-school chic through and through, with a hand-carved historical ceiling, leather armchairs and Damian Hirst paintings dotted around.

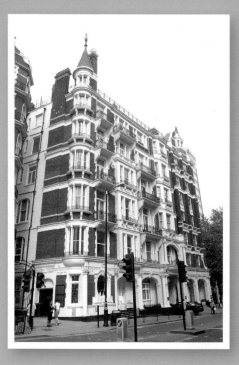

When a celebrity first-timer stops by the Wellington, a bottle with their name on is placed in a glass cupboard; it's now stocking the likes of Kate Moss, Jude Law, Bono and Mick Jagger.

For her twenty-sixth birthday, Cheryl decided to celebrate in Vanilla, a white minimalist venue with frosted mirrors and contemporary cascade chandeliers. The party was attended by her *X Factor* colleagues Simon Cowell, Louis Walsh, Dannii Minogue and Holly Willoughby.

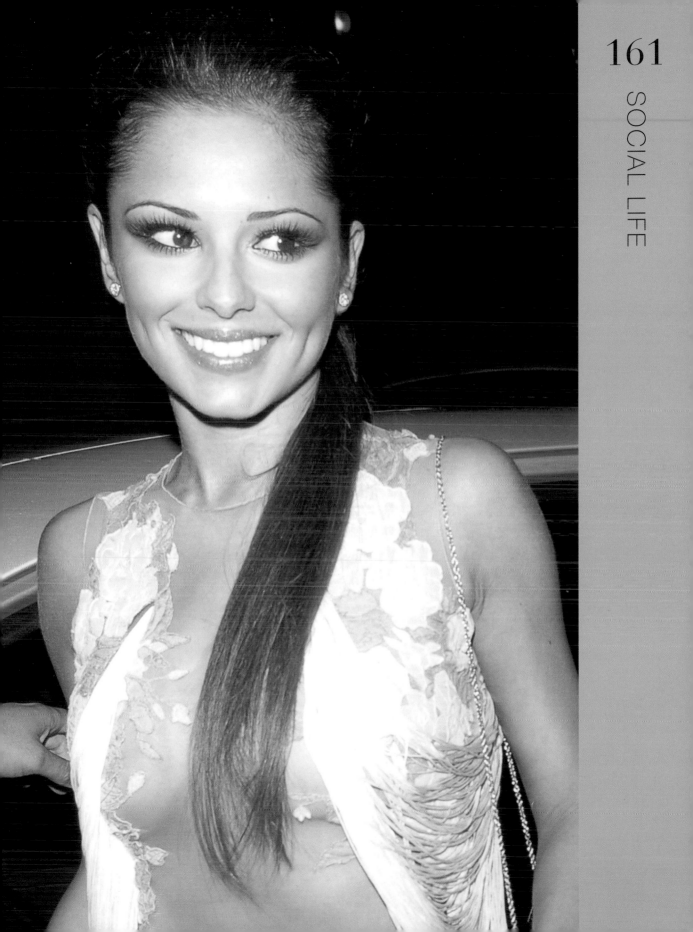

SOCIALIZING STATESIDE

Now that she's spending more time in LA, Cheryl has enjoyed going out on the town there, and has stopped by the Voyeur club on Santa Monica Boulevard with Derek Hough.

The club is an exclusive and sexy new hotspot with a burlesque flavour – provocative live art installations, pornographic wallpaper, live performances and sugar-free cocktails. Heidi Klum had her Halloween party there shortly after it opened and it has since become a favourite with the girls from *The Hills*, Justin Timberlake and Lindsay Lohan.

CLEAN LIVING

Even though Cheryl and her Girls Aloud bandmates got a reputation for wild partying when they first became famous, Cheryl openly admits that it was never really her scene. She is more of a homebody than a party girl, and although she still likes to kick up her heels and put on her glad rags for a night out with friends, you won't find her tumbling off her Louboutins any more.

Addiction in her family while she was growing up has shaped the way she feels about recreational drinking, as well as inspiring her strong anti-drugs stance. She told *Elle* she had first been put off drinking by her grandad, whom she says was killed by his addiction to booze, adding, 'It affected his kidneys and his mind. Drinking is scary to me now.'

Cheryl also doesn't touch drugs – and is scathing of those who do – after she had to live through the pain of having a heroin-addict boyfriend, a brother addicted to glue, and a childhood friend who died from a drugs overdose.

When Piers Morgan interviewed her for *GQ*, she cried uncontrollably when she recounted what had happened to some of the people closest to her, saying, 'It just broke my heart to see friends and family going through drugs. It put me off for life ...

'Where I come from, everyone is exposed to drugs and dealers. I'm just glad I was strong enough to resist it.'

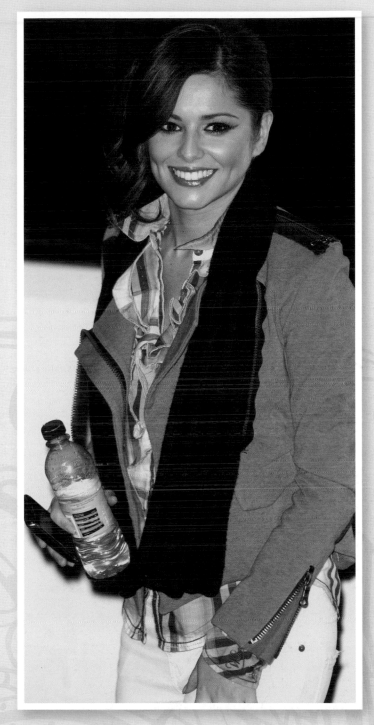

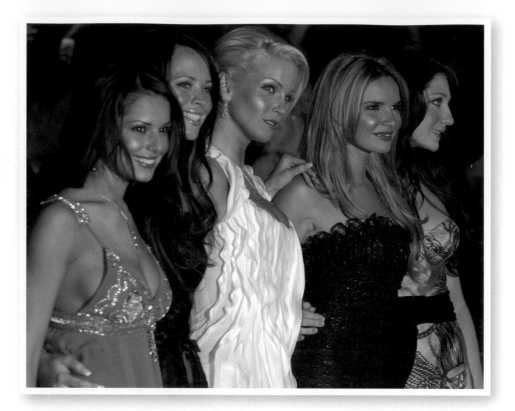

BEHIND THE VELVET ROPE

In the early days of Girls Aloud, Cheryl, all of a sudden, found herself invited to the most glamorous events imaginable. The excitement of walking the red carpet in a gorgeous dress in London's West End was like a surreal dream.

She went to a couple of premieres – Ant and Dec's comedy *Alien Autopsy* and romcom *It's a Boy Girl Thing* – but swiftly realized that premieres are basically just going to the cinema, but with a crowd of shouting people outside and photographers taking pictures.

The novelty wore off – and she was also wary of becoming one of the rent-a-celebs who turn up to the opening of an envelope, just to have their picture in the papers.

WORK IT

Wisely, Cheryl has been careful not to spread herself too thin ever since then, and now attends big showbiz bashes only if she is directly involved.

So she walked the red carpet with her girls for the premieres of *Love Actually* and *St Trinian's* – as they provided songs for the soundtracks – and she has also done her showbiz duty at the BRITs and the National Television Awards when she has been nominated with Girls Aloud or her *X Factor* colleagues.

These events are more PR than down time, though – and Cheryl treats them very much as 'on-duty' engagements, rather than as key moments in her social calendar.

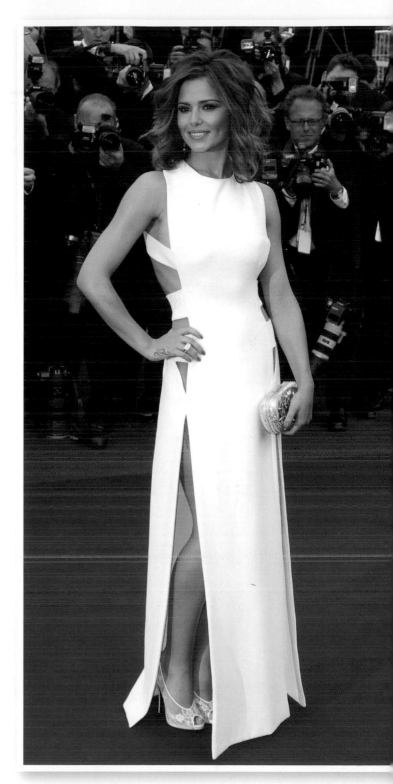

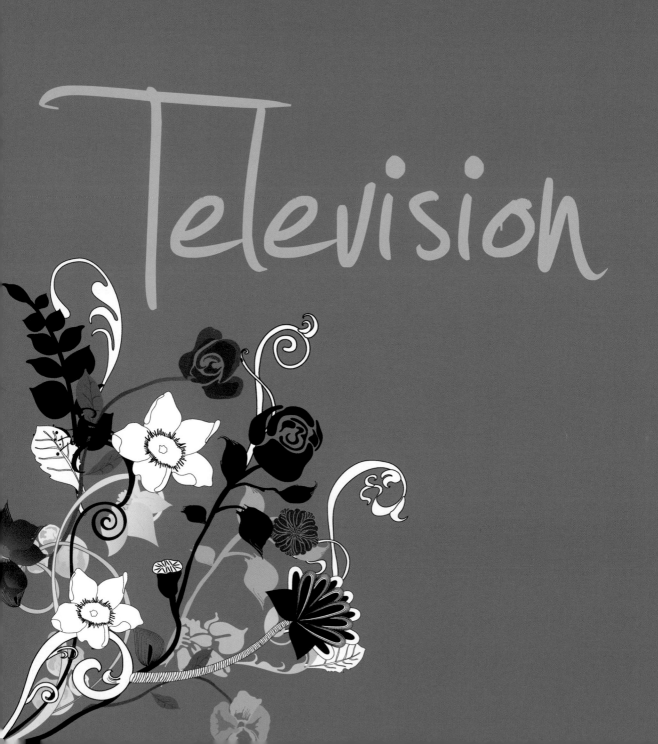

Television

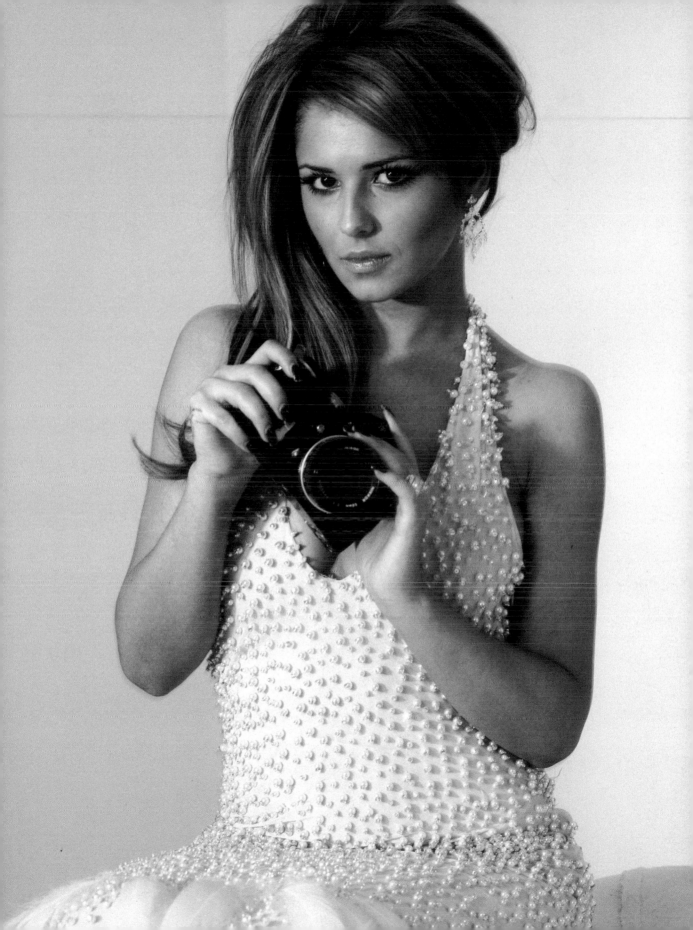

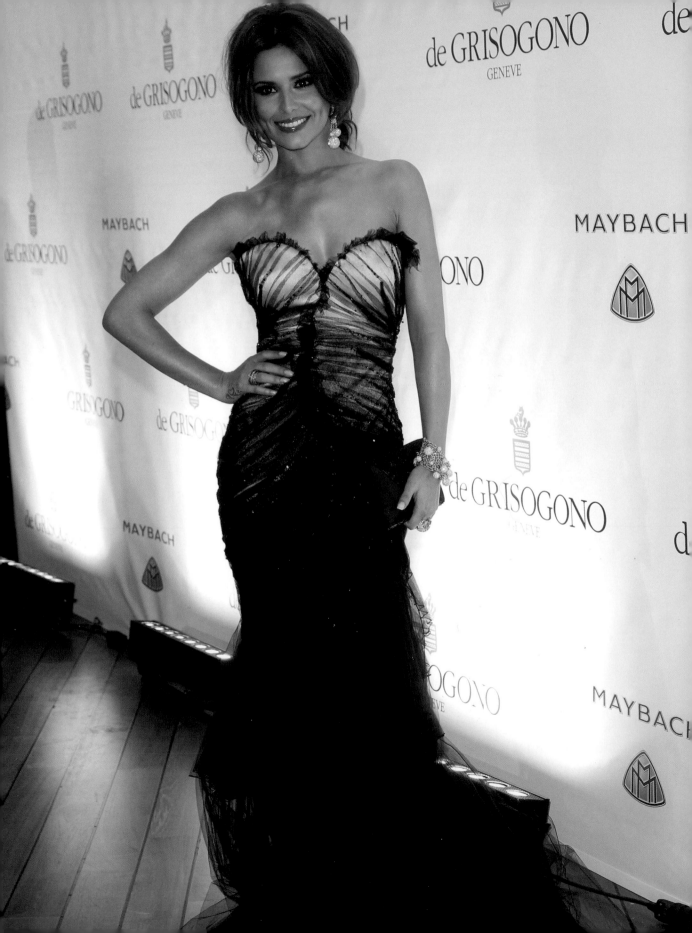

Cheryl has always stated very firmly that she is, first and foremost, a singer. She's never had a burning desire to diversify into presenting or acting – and yet her career has been intertwined with television ever since Pete Waterman mimed picking his jaw up off the floor after she sang S Club 7's 'Have You Ever' for her first audition on *Popstars: The Rivals.*

It would probably be fair to say that Cheryl doesn't have the cast-iron confidence that it takes to be a television presenter, but she is much more suited to the vehicles she's chosen, where she is followed by cameras as she interacts with others and has a chance to show viewers the 'real' her.

She does, however, have an ambitious nature, and ever since she was a little girl, growing up on a rough and poverty-stricken council estate, she has worked hard at becoming a success. She's a grafter, and that means she has embraced many career opportunities that have come her way, even though she may not have actively sought them out.

When she took part in *Comic Relief Does The Apprentice*, Sir Alan Sugar noticed her business potential, telling WENN, 'Cheryl Cole was very impressive. Everyone was expecting this dolly bird, but she showed street smarts, determination, great commitment and a very impressive business acumen. She'll go far, that girl.'

CHERYL'S PASSION

With Girls Aloud, Cheryl has made several TV programmes – a couple of fly-on-the-wall documentaries and a variety show – but the project of which she is most proud is probably *The Passions of … Girls Aloud*.

As the band matured, so did their desire to learn about things outside of their usual sphere of experience and so, in 2007, they signed up for the slightly left-field *Passions*, in which each girl was filmed learning a new skill.

Cheryl, who has always had a passion for all forms of dance, and who knows how to handle herself in tough surroundings, decided to learn how to krump – the street dance made popular in South Central, a rough area of LA, where she went to finish her training.

The process was a ferocious baptism of fire. Best friend Kimberley Walsh told the cameras, 'She's very self-critical,' and sure enough Cheryl was shown in tears during the challenging experience, sobbing, 'That's what the world will see. A heap of shit,' as she suffered a major moment of self-doubt.

Yet she came through – and then some. The final part of her training was to audition for a part in one of Will.i.am's videos. He was so impressed with her performance that he promoted her from backing dancer to guest vocals on his track 'Heartbreaker' – and the rest, as they say, is history.

Cheryl has tried her hand at TV presenting just three times, co-presenting *CD:UK* with Dave Berry in 2005, guest-presenting *The Friday Night Project* along with Kimberley and Sarah Harding in 2006, and taking the helm with all the girls for *The Friday Night Project* Christmas special in 2007.

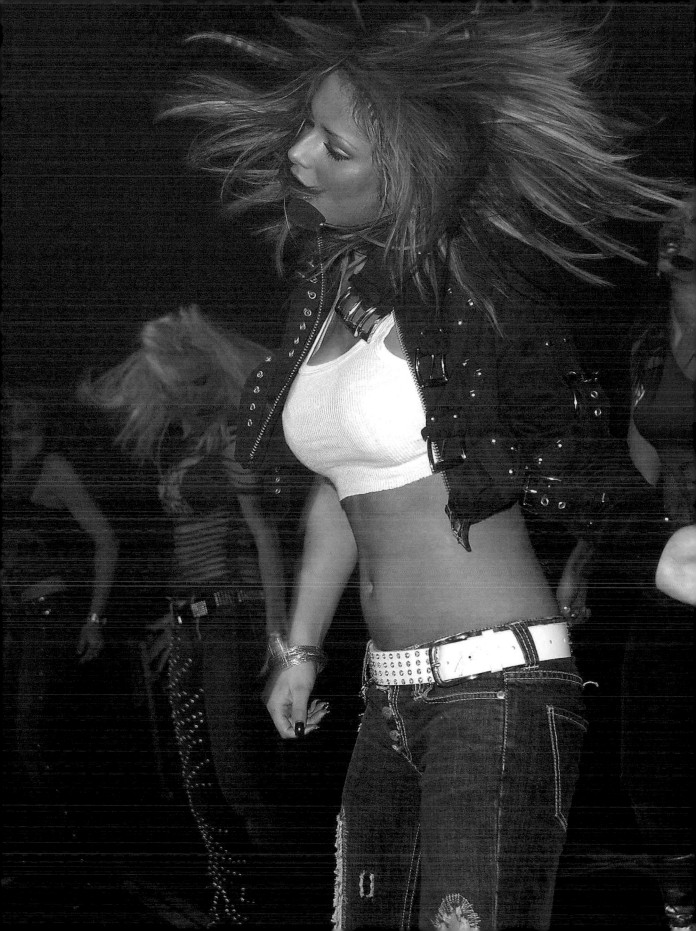

FAMILY VIEWING

With 10 million – plus – viewers tuning in to *The X Factor*, Cheryl was understandably nervous about such a major TV job. After her first broadcast, she was keen to get reassurance that she'd done OK. As she explained to *Attitude* magazine, 'I was waiting for a text or a call from me friends and family. But nothing. I was really hurt. So, after a long while, I texted my mother, saying, "Did you watch the show?" and she sent back: "Yes." That was it. "Yes"!'

Mum and daughter are so close, however, that Cheryl can say this with a smile on her face!

MAGIC MENTOR

Early in her first series, Cheryl set a precedent as to what kind of judge she was going to be when she was confronted with contestant Nikk Mager, whom she knew from when they were both trying to make it on *Popstars*. While Cheryl made it into Girls Aloud, Nikk was still slogging away trying to get a break.

Cheryl broke down in tears and walked out of his audition, refusing to judge him, but he was given a no from the other judges. Cheryl was devastated to be unable to help him when they had started out in exactly the same way.

Later, she crossed the line between judge and hopeful when she joined Aimee Buck onstage. The young girl had faltered after Simon said she wasn't good enough, so Cheryl duetted with her until she regained her composure.

> Cheryl has a flawless track record on *The X Factor*, winning the competition in both 2008 and 2009. She is the only judge to have won consecutively since the contest began.

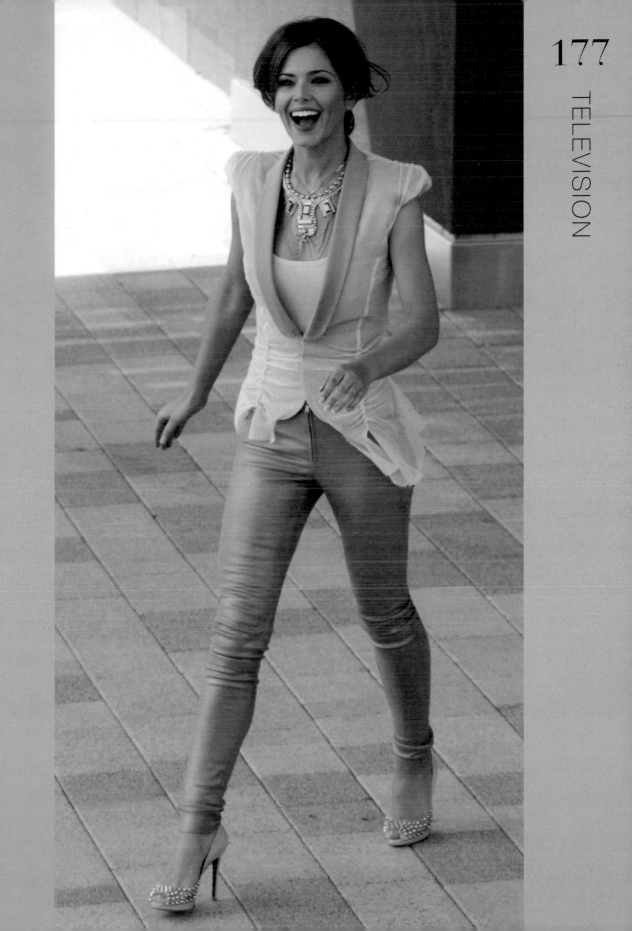

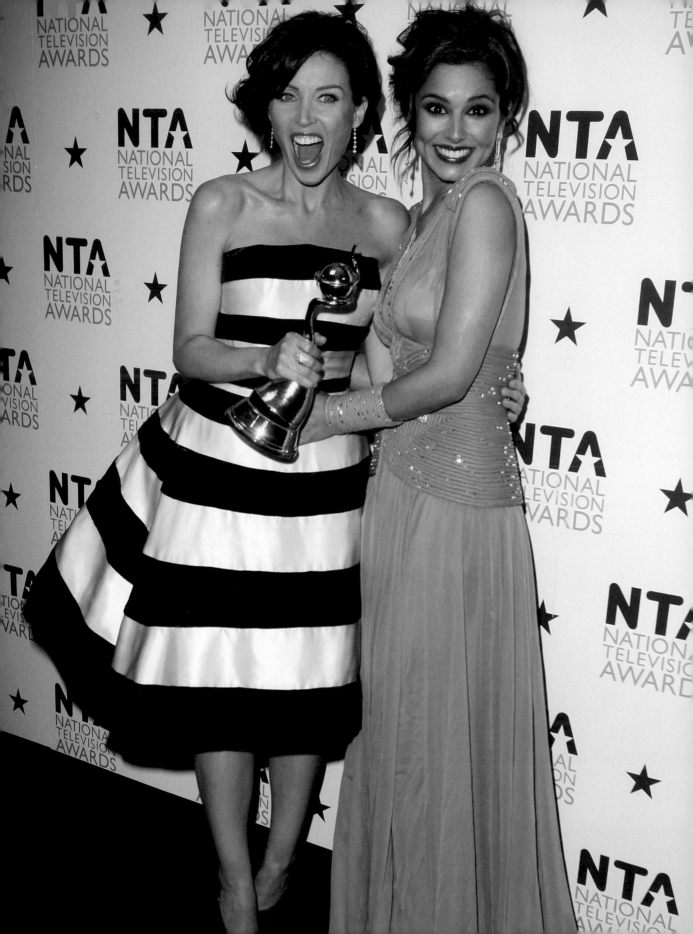

WORKING RELATIONSHIPS

When it comes to *The X Factor*, as much attention is given to the judges' relationships as to the contestants' talent. Cheryl and fellow judge Dannii Minogue have often been pitted against each other in the press, but – while they have both admitted they are not the closest of friends – they do genuinely get on.

As for Louis Walsh, who judged Cheryl when she was in *Popstars* and whom Girls Aloud had previously slated (because he was meant to be their manager, but was never around) – well, they have put their differences behind them. Cheryl told the *Mirror*, 'I've had a few run-ins with Louis. We both have strong opinions about what we believe in and that always makes for a few rows. But outside the show we have a brilliant friendship.'

And, despite her well-documented closeness to Simon, she explained to BBC News that, once it came to the competition, the love-in between them was off, saying, 'There is tension between us on the actual Saturday night, when he starts getting annoying and saying nasty things. It gets really heated backstage, and quite competitive.'

'It gets really heated backstage, and quite competitive.' BBC News

GOING SOLO

Just after launching her solo music career, Cheryl was given her own Saturday night TV show, *Cheryl Cole's Night In*, which aired between two episodes of *The X Factor* during peak December scheduling. The programme featured her performing and being interviewed by Holly Willoughby, as well as performances from Rihanna, Alexandra Burke, Will Young, Snow Patrol and her old buddy Will.i.am.

It was a similar project to the Girls Aloud Christmas variety show, *The Girls Aloud Party*, which had aired the year before.

Cheryl showed her sense of humour on *The Girls Aloud Party*, featuring in several self-deprecating comedy sketches, including one where she and best buddy Kimberley dressed up as old women gossiping about old times.

In 2009, Cheryl was on her own. Her own TV show, with her own name in the title, and the focus all on her.

It was a very significant sign of how her TV career is progressing – and of the high esteem in which she is held by broadcasters. As far as the future of Cheryl's TV career is concerned ... the sky's the limit.

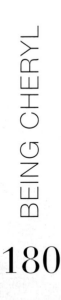
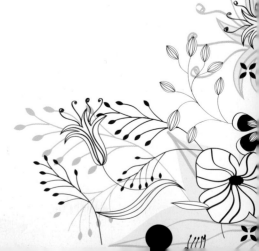

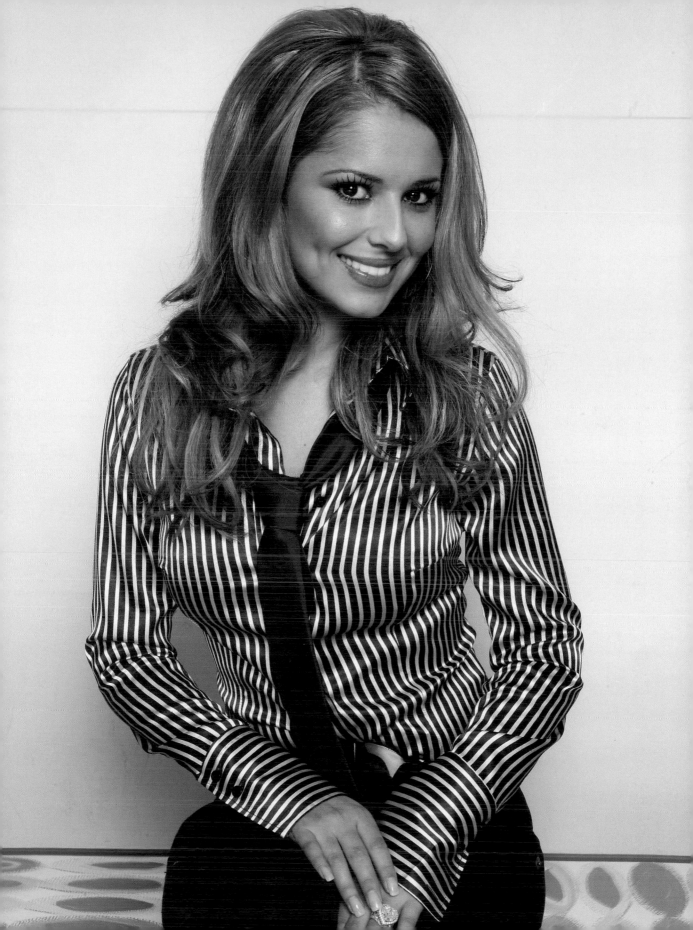

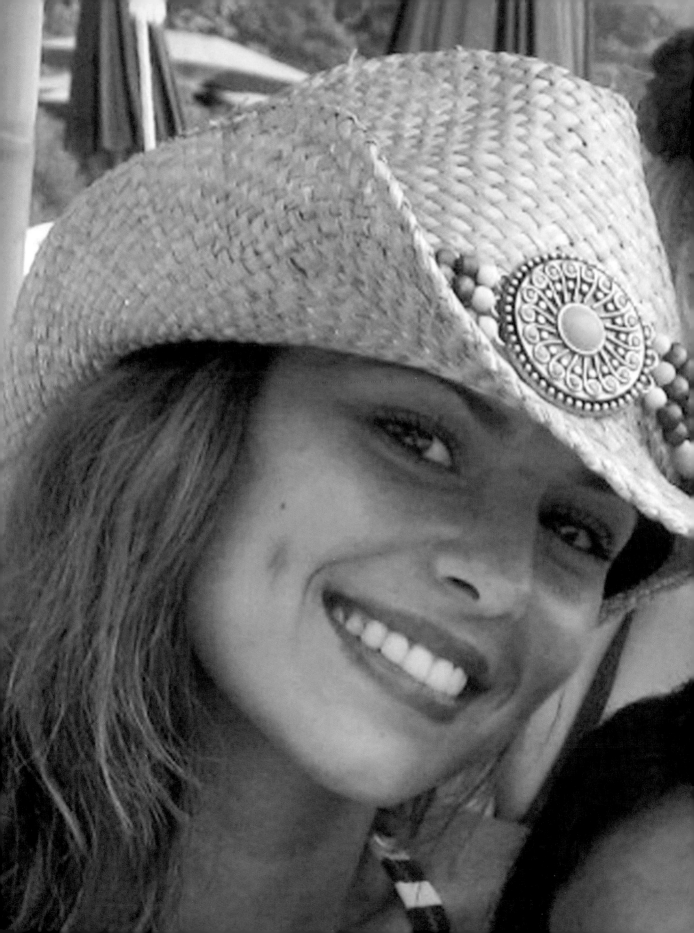

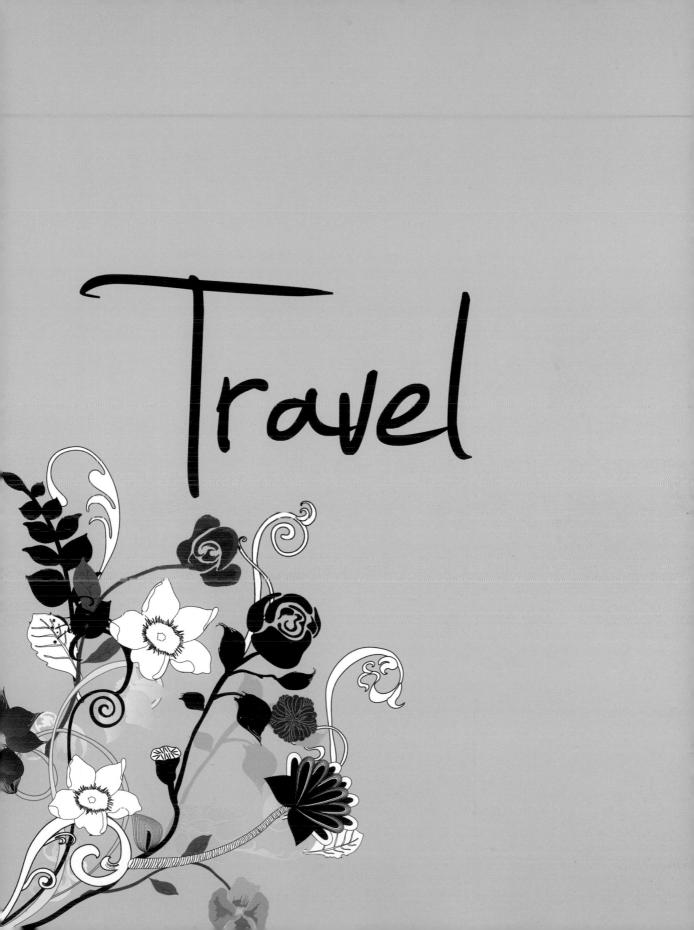

Travel

When a pop star travels overseas, it's all about five-star accommodation with walk-in shoe closets, private jets and luxury yachts. However, the ones who work for their lifestyle are usually so busy that they don't have time for their days to turn into one long holiday – although they certainly make up for it when they do get a break.

Cheryl travels all over Europe and the States for her career, but for the most part she has mainly been on only one holiday a year since Girls Aloud took off.

She always heads for the sun and while some celebrities go to the same place time and time again – like Simon Cowell and his beloved Barbados – she has travelled all over the world, exploring the Indian Ocean, the Caribbean and Europe, but not often returning to the same location.

Patriotic Cheryl still says that Newcastle is one of her favourite places in the world. She takes a little piece of home with her wherever she goes – according to *People* magazine, she always checks in under the pseudonym 'Miss England'.

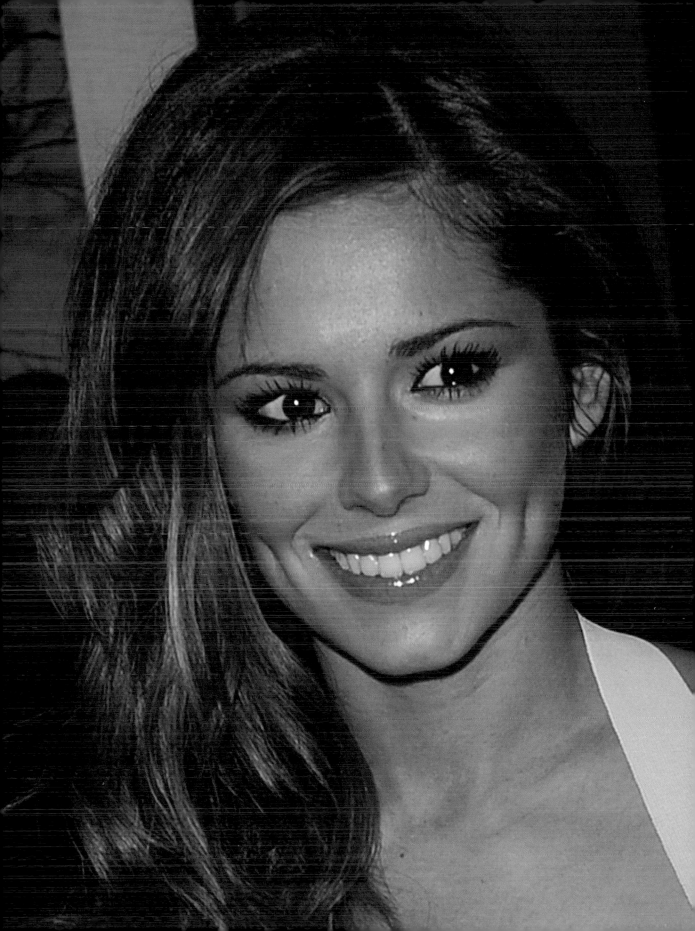

GET HER HOLIDAY LOOK

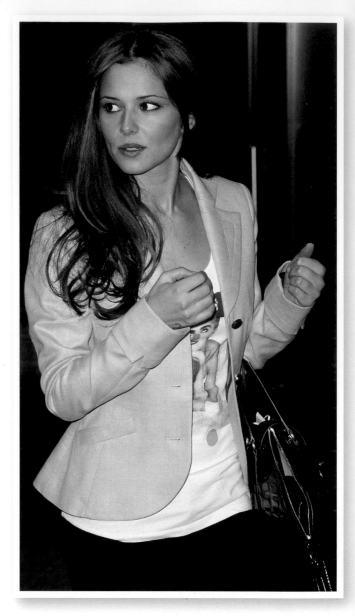

AT THE AIRPORT

Over the years, Cheryl has become queen of the airport outfit – only Victoria Beckham rivals her in the amount of times they are snapped going through arrivals or departures.

Like Victoria, Cheryl is always immaculate, favouring skinny jeans, skyscraper heels, a funky vest or T-shirt, fitted jackets, the obligatory big handbag and long necklaces.

AIRPORT STYLE

★ Skinny jeans
★ Towering high heels
★ Long necklaces or a scarf
★ Funky T-shirts
★ Fitted jackets
★ Designer handbags

ON FOREIGN SHORES

Once Cheryl reaches her destination, it's all about comfort – although always still with a little bit of bling. She opts for animal prints, dangling charms, jewelled swimming costumes and a trusty straw cowboy hat for all occasions.

'I've got loads of bits that I bring out for holiday,' Cheryl told *OK!* magazine. 'I do love a kaftan for when it gets a bit chilly and I love maxi dresses. They're brilliant if you've overdone it by the beach with the chips; they hide a multitude of sins. I always have a couple of those bad boys in the wardrobe.'

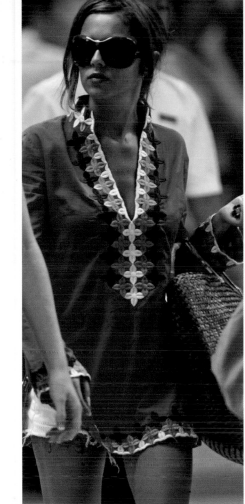

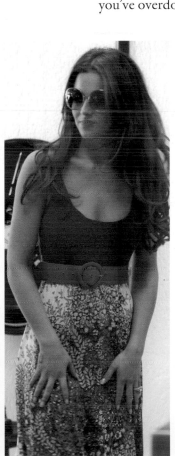

When she travels, Cheryl always has with her a tube of all-round favourite-of-the-stars Elizabeth Arden Eight Hour Cream, which multi-tasks as a lip balm, intensive hand cream and moisturizer for dry skin.

BEATING JET LAG

With all her transatlantic travel, Cheryl has become a dab hand at beating energy-sapping jet lag. She shared her expertise with *Stylist*, saying, 'You have to have a plan in your head when you're going to sleep on the plane and what time you'll get up. If you're not strict, you'll just feel like death for a week.'

CHERYL'S FAVOURITE DESTINATIONS

- ★ LA
- ★ Thailand
- ★ Marbella
- ★ Newcastle!

JET-SET DESTINATIONS

Cheryl has travelled the globe on her various holidays. Though she's picked out certain destinations she loves, it's clear that her adventurous side is still exploring and experimenting. Here's a rundown of just a few of the hotspots she's taken in on her tour of the world's most glamorous locations.

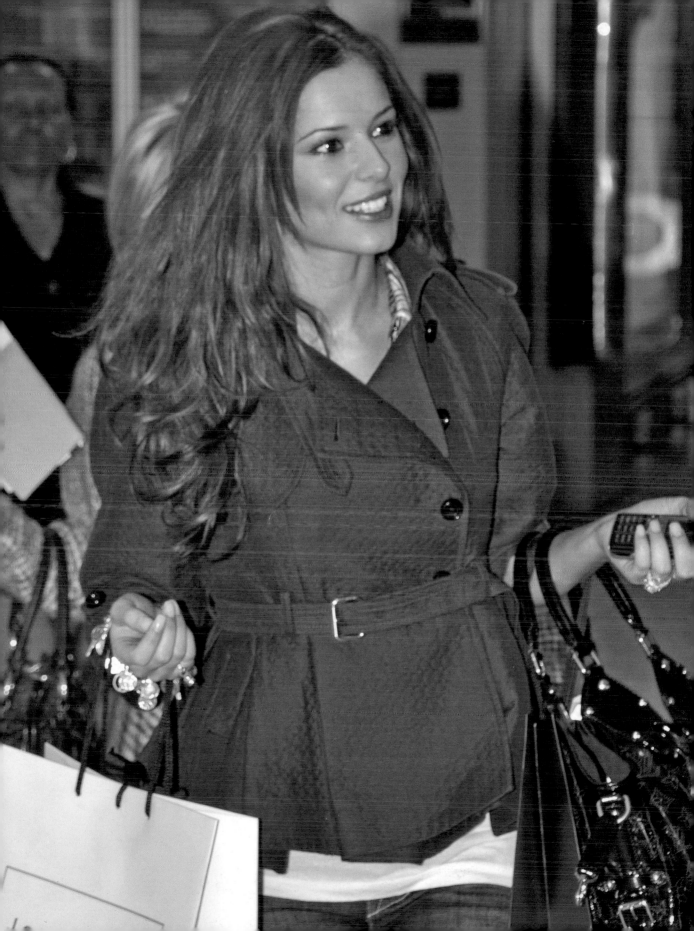

DUBAI

Cheryl likes a lively atmosphere on holiday and in 2005 she and Ashley headed off to Dubai in the United Arab Emirates to celebrate the end of the football season.

> Dubai is a hugely popular destination with Brits as it takes less than seven hours to get there and is a haven of perfectly manufactured beaches, year-round sunshine, luxury resorts and air-conditioned shopping malls.

Dubai has traditionally been a favourite of footballers, with John and Toni Terry, Peter Crouch and Abbey Clancy, and Cristiano Ronaldo all visiting; while the Beckhams and Brad Pitt and Angelina Jolie have bought properties in the mind-bogglingly exclusive Palm Jumeirah, comprised of a string of artificial islands.

Cheryl stayed in a villa, but didn't just spend her time idling by the pool: she got stuck into the local activities and did some exploring. She went off into the desert for a safari in a golf buggy and also took a camel ride.

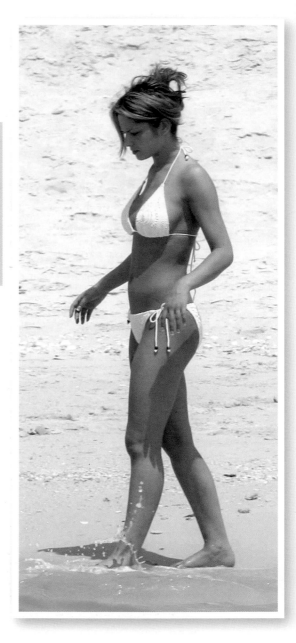

MARBELLA

The flashy Spanish region that has been dubbed the Spanish Riviera is one of the only holiday destinations Cheryl has returned to; she has visited at least three times for her summer vacations.

She has always favoured the luxury resort of Puerto Banus – a marina town that plays host to multi-million-pound yachts and is rammed with designer shops, which has led to it becoming known as southern Spain's answer to St Tropez.

She went there for the first time with Ashley, after they got back from Dubai. The couple stayed at The Ocean Club, which is a party hotspot – young and trendy with contemporary décor and one of the biggest swimming pools in Europe: a huge oval, which has expansive circular white leather beds in the VIP area.

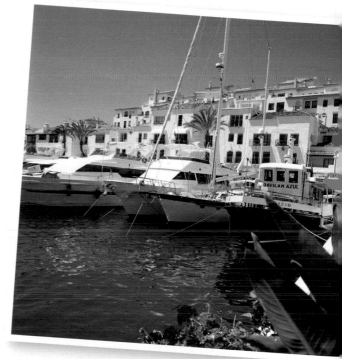

When they returned two years later, Cheryl was photographed drinking rosé wine and champagne; they also returned after the first set of troubles in 2008, and were snapped walking down the beach together drinking cocktails.

Although many celebrities like to get on the tropical property ladder, buying homes in luxury destinations, Cheryl is yet to invest in a holiday retreat, preferring to stay in hotels and villas.

THE SEYCHELLES

For the likes of Salma Hayek and François-Henri Pinault, Brad Pitt and Jennifer Aniston, and Elizabeth Hurley and Arun Nayar, all of whom honeymooned in the Seychelles, it may have been a paradise island away from the noise and chatter of funkier tropical hotspots like St Barths or Miami – but for Cheryl and Ashley on their honeymoon in 2006, it was a different matter, as they found the island too quiet!

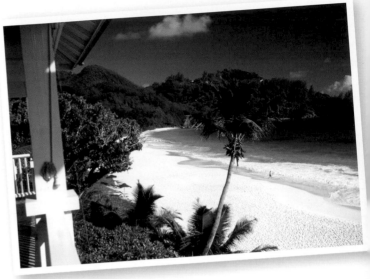

After hearing rumours that she was looking to buy a holiday home there, Cheryl told *The Sun*, 'It's rubbish. We went there for our honeymoon and it was the most boring place ever.'

The remote Seychelles are a chain of islands in the Indian Ocean off the east coast of Africa. They are a top favourite with celebrities because of the amount of private islands, which means photographers can't take unauthorized pictures.

The downside for Cheryl was the lack of nightlife. She stayed in the Banyan Tree on the main island of Mahe, which was rich with luxuries like a private butler, private beach and palm tree garden – but while it might be the ideal place for those in the public eye to disappear, it's obviously not for those who are used to the bright lights and funky music of Marbella.

BARBADOS

This ultra-luxurious Caribbean island is a favourite of Beyoncé and Jay-Z, Jennifer Aniston, Hugh Grant, Davina McCall and Barbadian-born Rihanna. Cheryl headed off to the island's premier resort Sandy Lane (pictured) in June 2007.

Barbados is probably one of the most popular and well-known tourist destinations in the Caribbean and the west coast is gilded with exclusive resorts. It's where Simon Cowell is spotted sailing and jet-skiing every New Year, and many, like him, visit annually for their Christmas break.

Sandy Lane is the jewel in the crown, with multi-spray showers, make-up rooms and private verandahs. One of the house specialities is Bajan fish balls, which was a treat for seafood fan Cheryl.

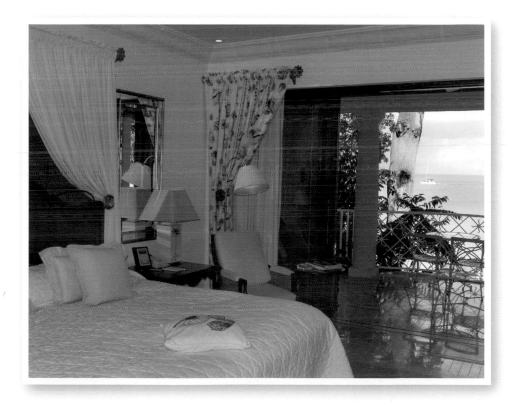

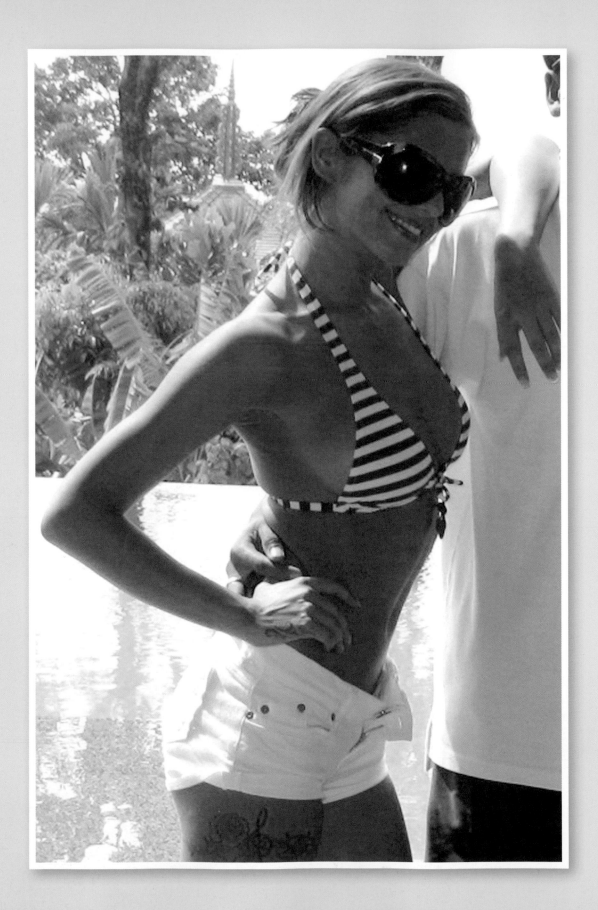

THAILAND

Although the correct pronunciation of the famous Thai resort is 'puh-ket', it seems to be more than coincidence that the notoriously feisty Cheryl, Kimberley and Nicola chose to holiday in the destination Phuket after the allegations about Ashley cheating on Cheryl early in 2008.

Cheryl took off with her two best friends and enjoyed a girlie vacation in the Trisara resort, which has villas with private gardens and infinity pools; the restaurants specialize in seafood and curries.

Cheryl told the *Mirror* when she got back, 'The holiday was fantastic, just what I needed,' while Nicola added that they spent their whole time chatting, sunbathing and drinking cocktails, adding in *OK!*, 'We had such a relaxing time. It was nice to get away and we really had such a laugh.'

The country must have made an impression as Cheryl listed it as one of her favourite places in *Dreams That Glitter*, adding, 'Thailand's a beautiful place and the people are really nice.'

'Thailand's a beautiful place.'

Dreams That Glitter

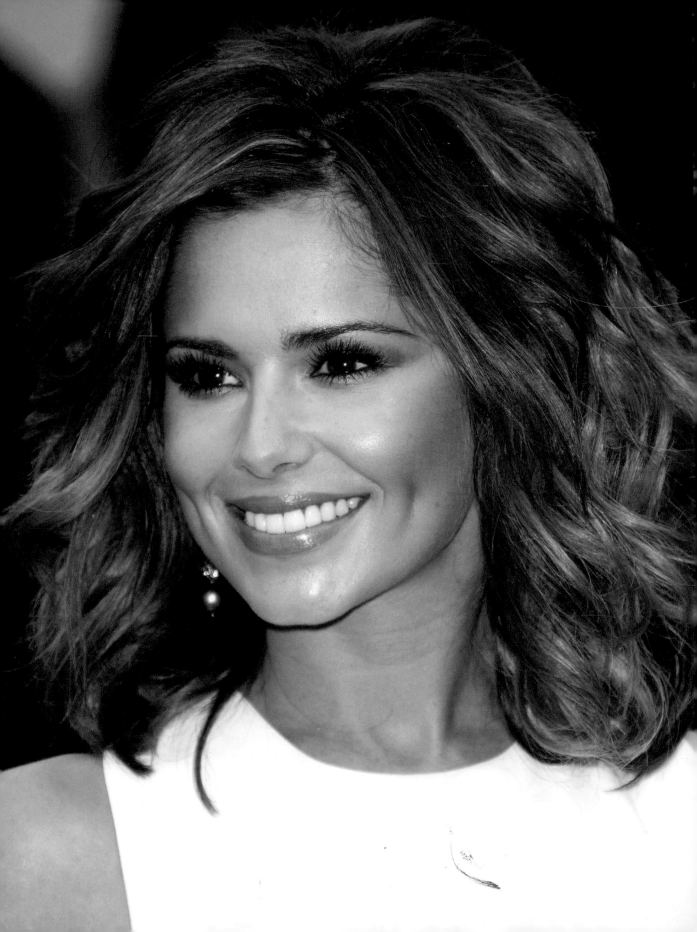

THE FRENCH RIVIERA

Cheryl has also spent time soaking up the sun on the French Riviera. Following in the footsteps of Hollywood starlets and home-grown celebs alike, in the summer of 2009 she visited the area for a sunshine break, staying on Chelsea boss Roman Abramovich's yacht.

She returned to the area in summer 2010, mixing business with pleasure as she performed at a party in Antibes hosted by luxury jewellery company de Grisogono at the glamorous Hôtel du Cap, and then later joined her pal Will.i.am in the DJ booth as the pair partied into the night. In the same trip, she made a scene-stealing appearance at the Cannes Film Festival, wowing film buffs and fashionistas alike as she worked the red carpet in a daring white Versace gown with cutout panels and a thigh-high slit.

CAPE TOWN

In December 2009, Cheryl headed to the South African city with her mum. After working solidly throughout the autumn promoting her debut album, as well as filming *The X Factor*, she was more than ready for a break.

She made the most of the winter sun at the exclusive Clifton Beach, which is next to Table Mountain and renowned for its exceptionally high quality white sandy beaches. They have even achieved blue flag status, which is reserved for only the best quality beaches on the planet.

Of course, it wasn't all about the relaxing and sunbathing, as Cheryl likes the contrast of a lively nightlife as well. On 31 December, she was a guest of US businessman Preston Haskell, who owns a vineyard out there, at his fabulous New Year's Eve party.

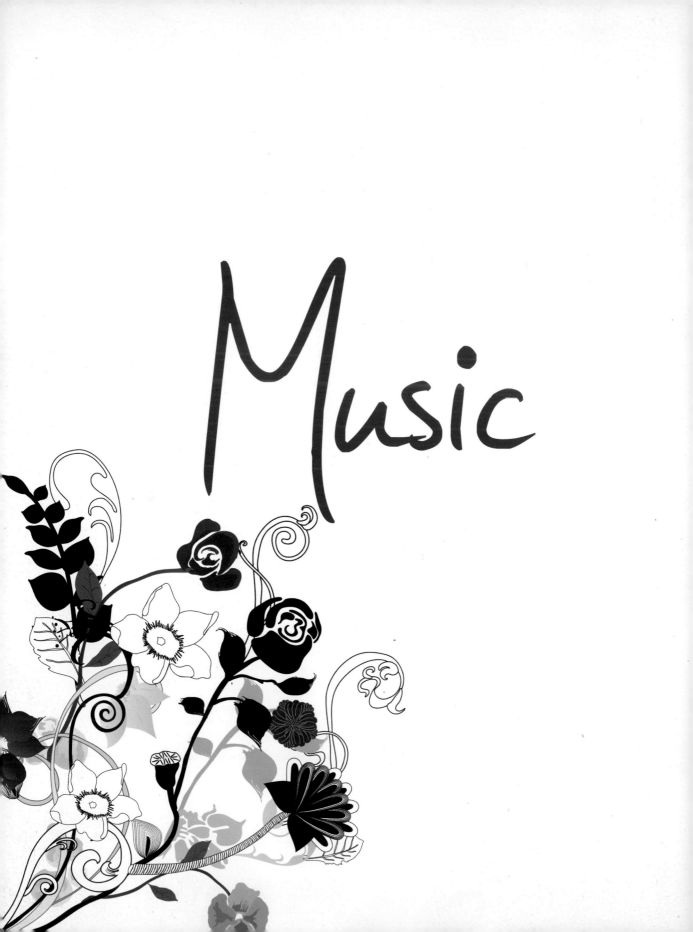

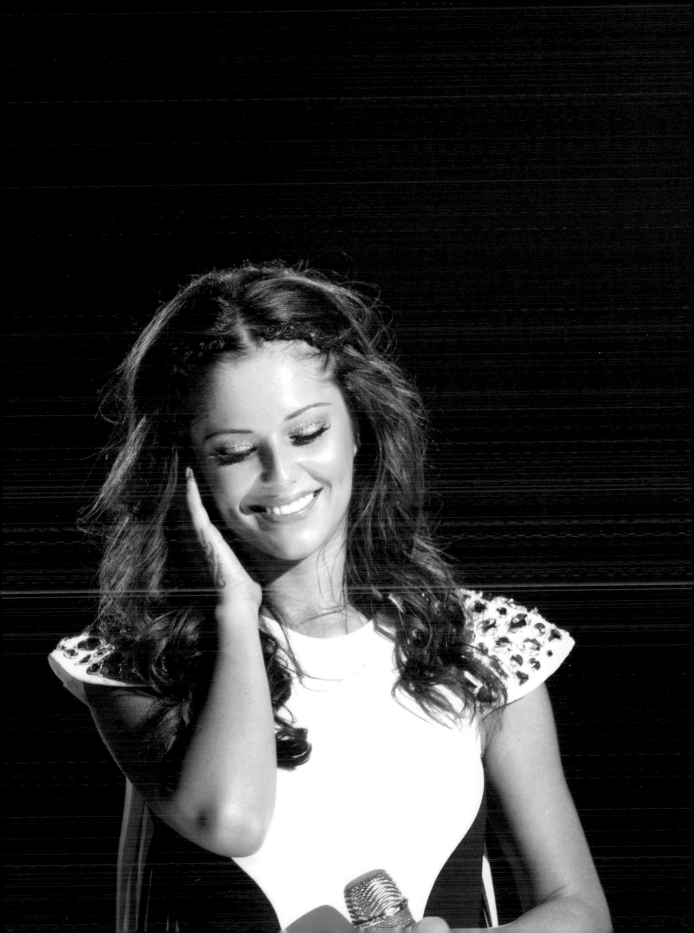

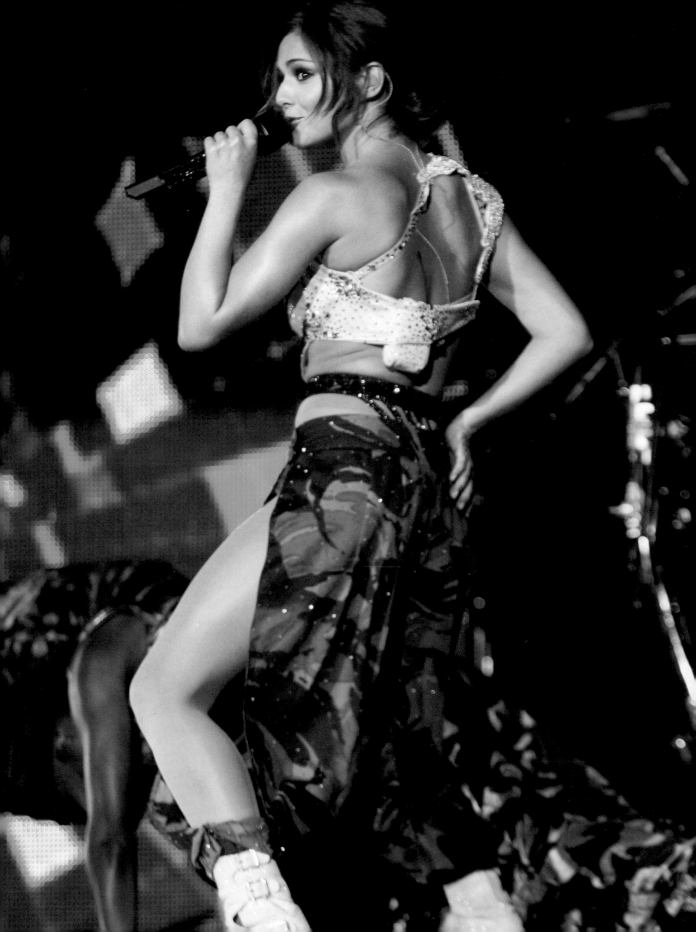

With so much focus on Cheryl's TV career, style choices, haircuts, friendships and relationship issues, it could be easy to forget that what she is, first and foremost, is a pop singer.

She has wanted to sing, dance and entertain for as long as she can remember, and over the years she and her bandmates have become the most successful girl group of all time, shooting into the *Guinness Book of Records* in a blaze of sequins and sass.

The costumes, make-up, lights, sets and backing dancers are all important parts of the world of pop, but they would all be for nothing if the beat didn't make people want to dance, the melody didn't leave people singing to themselves, and the music didn't just simply make people feel better.

And now Cheryl is taking all she has learned along the way and flying high in her solo career, with her debut single and album both going to number one.

THE NEW POP ROYALTY

Ever since the unforgettably exciting discordant jangling of debut single 'Sound of the Underground', Cheryl has been a musical force to be reckoned with.

At first, she and Girls Aloud were written off as Spice Girls wannabes and reality-show one-hit wonders, but they swiftly proved that as well as being feisty, intelligent and talented, they could produce some of the best and most successful pop music in history.

The Spice Girls ruled the airwaves for just four years; Girls Aloud have been striding over the pop landscape in their towering Louboutins for more than twice as long. In that time, they have racked up six platinum albums and twenty consecutive top-ten singles – the most ever for a girl group; knocking Destiny's Child, who were the previous record-holders with a somewhat paltry eleven, off the number-one slot.

BREAKING THE RULES

From the beginning, Girls Aloud were more than just the archetypal pop puppets being jerked around at the end of a gilded chain – they were five young women in control of their lives.

Despite landing a record contract with a major company, they were given no guidance about how to survive in the industry, and got through the first few

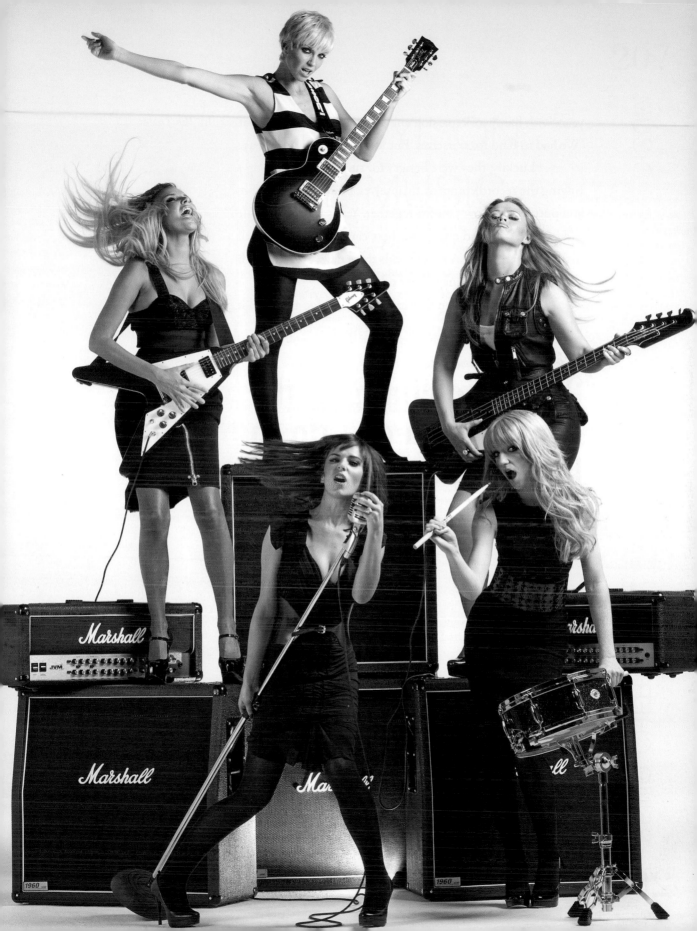

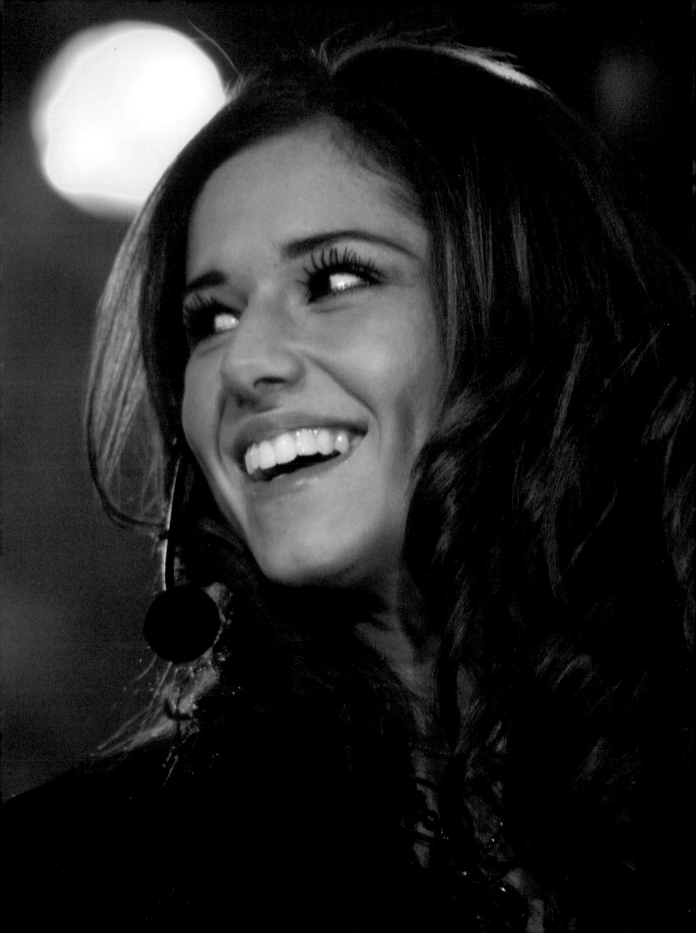

TASTE IN MUSIC

Music is one of the greatest pleasures in Cheryl's life. She is, first and foremost, an R & B and soul girl, which are the genres of music she grew up listening to.

Her favourite artists are Mary J. Blige, Beyoncé and Alicia Keys; she walked down the aisle to Alicia Keys's 'If I Ain't Got You'. John Legend is another favourite: she and Ashley went to see him in concert for one of their first dates, and Cheryl later flew the soul singer over from the States as Ashley's wedding present, so Legend could perform 'Stay with You' for their first dance.

However, it's Beyoncé who gets her ultimate respect: in a live web chat with fans, Cheryl said that if she could listen to only one artist for the rest of her life, it would be Beyoncé. 'I think she would fulfil everything you need,' Cheryl explained. 'I love watching massive performances with all the dancing and pyrotechnics, she can do that, but she can also give you those spine-tingling ballad moments.'

CHERYL'S IDOLS

★ Beyoncé
★ Lady Gaga
★ John Legend
★ Alicia Keys
★ Mary J. Blige

INSPIRATION

Like many artists, Cheryl casts her net far and wide when it comes to being inspired on the musical front. On the indie side, she has said that 'Yellow' by Coldplay is one of her favourite songs, and she's a fan of Snow Patrol too.

Yet she also admires modern female artists, praising Kate Nash's 'Foundations' in the *Daily Star* – 'the lyrics are great: so well written' – commending Duffy's work – 'she has an amazing voice for someone so young. It's so pure' – and singling out her heroine Lady Gaga for particular acclamation, telling *FemaleFirst*, 'As a style icon and an artist, I'm slightly obsessed with her. She's the real deal.'

As you might expect, being one herself, Cheryl takes inspiration from pop divas too, saying how exciting it was to meet Britney Spears, whom she had always looked up to, and revealing how intimidating it was to perform on the same *X Factor* show as her idol Whitney Houston.

'I wouldn't get out of bed if music didn't exist. There'd be no point in living – I feel that strongly.' *Dreams That Glitter*

GOING IT ALONE

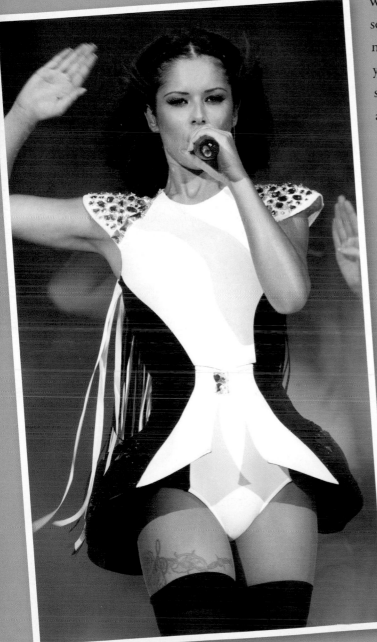

When it came to launching her solo career, Cheryl was incredibly nervous, even though she had eight years of experience. The seeds were sown almost by chance after she auditioned for Will.i.am as part of her street-dancing challenge for *The Passions of ... Girls Aloud*. The Black Eyed Peas frontman liked her and she ended up not just performing in his video, but also singing backing vocals.

Cheryl revealed to cherylcole.com that the duo then stayed in touch: 'We became friends and he said he was interested in working with me again. It was a massive compliment, but I didn't even register it, really. I was working hard with the girls. They were my complete focus.'

However, when the girls all determined to take some time off, she decided to go for it, and started working with Will over in LA.

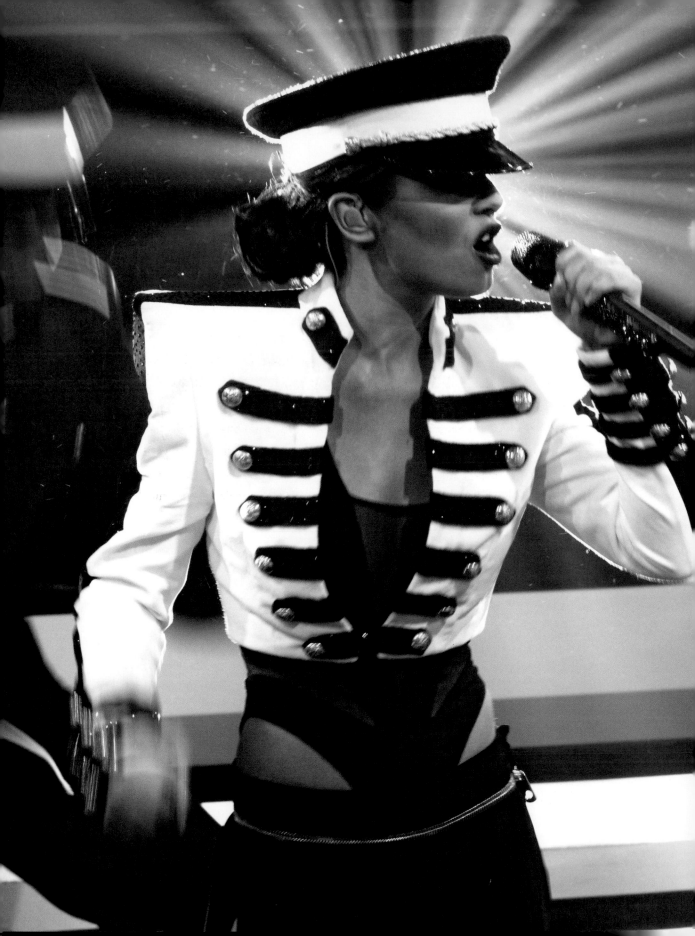

THE SOUND OF CHERYL

Sticking to her roots, Cheryl opted to create a hybrid of pop, dance and R & B for her debut record. She told cherylcole.com that the style of working with Will was different from working on Girls Aloud material, explaining that she had more of a say in the content.

'The way we work with Girls Aloud is that we'll go into the vocal booth and do our lines on a track that's already almost completed. With Will, I was seeing music being made right from the ground up. He'd ask my opinion on the beats and the words. He'd send me off to write hooks.'

Radio 1 DJ Scott Mills lavished praise on the resulting music in the *Mirror*, saying, 'If I was to describe her stuff in three words, I'd say sassy, cool and "now". Cheryl is doing amazingly well musically because she's working with all the right people who give her the cool edge lots of female pop stars struggle to achieve.'

'Cheryl's the girl of the moment in every way.'

Radio 1 DJ Scott Mills, *Mirror*

Cheryl's debut solo single went to number one, her first three singles all made the top five, and her debut solo album went to number one and was certified platinum.

SOLO STAR

In summer 2010, Cheryl toured with the Black Eyed Peas – but all that was a million miles away as she faced her first live solo performance: on *The X Factor*, in front of an audience of millions … and executed just metres from the judges' table, at which sat Simon Cowell.

She performed an energetic rendition of 'Fight for this Love' in her red-jacketed, military-inspired costume – and received a standing ovation from the judges. An impressed Simon saluted her.

Just a few weeks later, she wore a white version of the outfit for Children in Need – and cemented her growing reputation as an A-list solo star when she also performed a duet with indie rockers Snow Patrol.

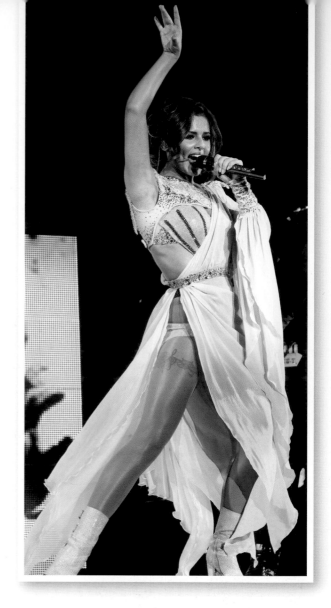

By the time she performed her anthemic number on *Cheryl Cole's Night In* – in hot pink with her backing dancers dressed as Samurai – she was really having fun!

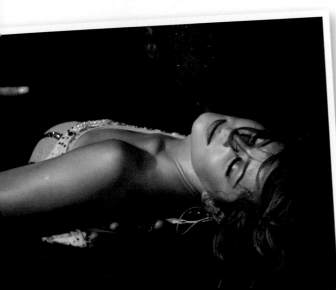

THE BRITS

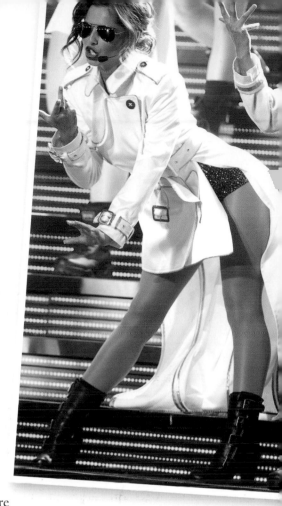

But just two months later, when she performed the same song again at the BRIT Awards, things were very different. She had recently split from Ashley and it marked the first time she had performed since the announcement. People were watching her every lip-glossed word.

    Cheryl didn't disappoint. The reworking of the performance was electric as she sprang up onto the stage from below and performed the first half of the number in a micro-mini white trench coat and aviators, surrounded by female dancers, before 'Fight for this Love' segued into Steve Angello's remix of the Robin S classic 'Show Me Love'.

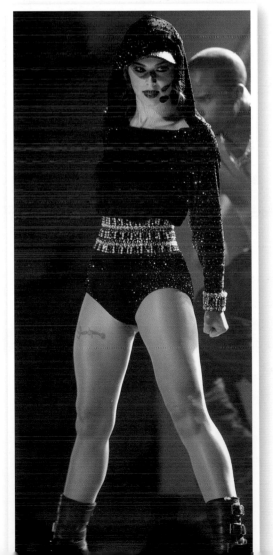

    For this section of the routine, Cheryl re-emerged in a black leotard and hood with a posse of topless men. Her dancing was strong, tough and powerful, with every gesture loaded with intensity and focus. The irony of the lyrics wasn't missed on anyone, but Cheryl carried it off with aplomb.

COMING TO AMERICA

With Cheryl spending more time in the States and befriending a number of US stars, speculation has been building about how much of a pop success she would be overseas, with Simon Cowell telling the *Mirror*, 'I think she'd be great over here – Cheryl's a star.'

Sharon Osbourne, who has now lived most of her life in the States and been part of the music industry for decades, knows what it takes, and told the *Mirror*, 'She's got a great career, she's sassy and approachable. She'll do brilliantly in America, they'll love her.'

Even Rihanna, who appeared on *Cheryl Cole's Night In*, has been confident enough about Cheryl breaking the States to speak publicly about it, telling the *Mirror*, 'Cheryl is cute and incredible. I'd love to have her on the tour, in Europe or in America. I think I could help break her into the States. She'd wow them.'

As for the lady herself, Cheryl told BBC Radio 1's Fearne Cotton, 'I love the thought of it and I would love to do it. The talent out there is phenomenal. I would buzz off them, but whether they would buzz off me, I don't know … but if the opportunity is there, I will give 110 per cent.'

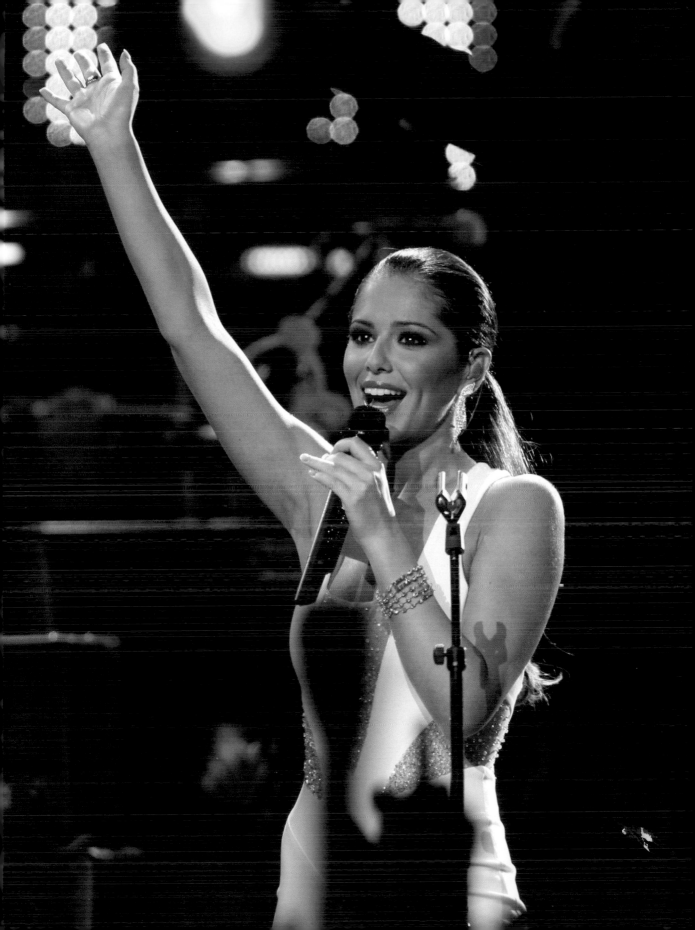

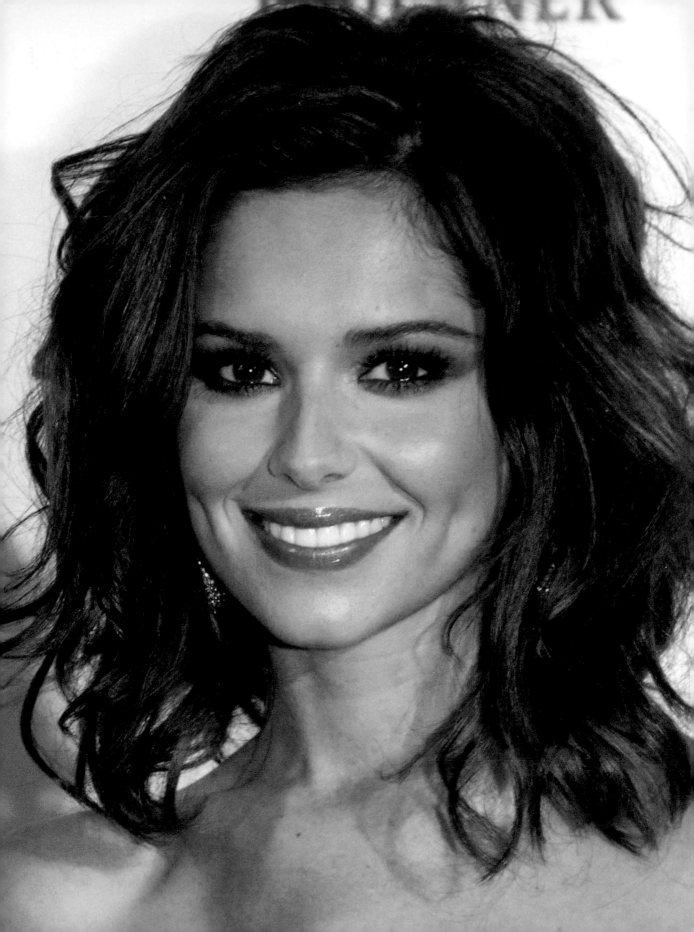

Being Cheryl

At the age of nineteen, when a desperately nervous and unpolished Cheryl first stepped into the spotlight, she could never have imagined the impact she would have on the British public – but that is exactly why she is so loved.

She has learned everything the hard way, genuinely learned from her mistakes and the things she has been through, and wants to use her experiences to help people, especially the next generation.

Her coffee-cream complexion, killer wardrobe and nice line in Simon Cowell put-downs are all much envied, and deservedly so, but there's more to the pop princess and Saturday night star than what you see on TV. Aspects of the nervous young girl who still bites her nails remain – and at the heart of the woman is the ambitious grafter who takes every opportunity with both hands and gives it her all.

After interviewing Cheryl, *Attitude* magazine summed her up perfectly, saying: 'During the interview, she switches gear from giggly to incandescent, teary to ecstatic, proud to just *so* grateful within the blink of an exquisitely mascara-ed lash. And every single sentiment is felt with absolute full-on ferocious conviction. If you ask her a question, she will answer it straight from the heart or direct from the gut.'

Cheryl is loved because she's emotional but strong, flawed but aspirational, professional but honest. There are a lot of dizzying highs and crashing lows in being Cheryl – but as long as she still has the glint in her eye and the fire in her belly, the designer handbag flung over her arm and the Louboutins on her size-five feet, she'll continue to capture our hearts. And that's what being Cheryl is all about.

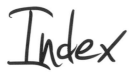

Index